Positive Health

Designs for Action

Positive Health
Designs for Action

Mary K. Beyrer, Ph.D.
Professor of Health Education,
The Ohio State University

Wesley P. Cushman, Ed.D.
Professor Emeritus, Health Education,
The Ohio State University

Robert Kaplan, Ph.D.
Professor of Health Education,
The Ohio State University

Marian K. Solleder, Ph.D.
Professor of Health Education,
University of North Carolina
   at Greensboro

Second Edition

LEA & FEBIGER   Philadelphia 1977

Health Education, Physical Education, and Recreation

RUTH ABERNATHY, Ph.D.

Editorial Adviser

Professor Emeritus, School of Physical and Health Education
University of Washington, Seattle 98105

Library of Congress Cataloging in Publication Data

Main entry under title:

Positive health : designs for action.

.(Health education, physical education, and recreation
series)
    Original ed., 1965 by W. P. Cushman and others.
    Includes index.
    SUMMARY: Discusses health problems facing young
adults, including sexuality, drugs, nutrition, disease,
and pollution.
    1. Hygiene. 2. Public health. [1. Hygiene.
2. Public health] I. Beyrer, Mary K. II. Cushman,
Wesley P. Positive health.
    RA776.C964 1977   613   76-22769

ISBN 0-8121-0572-9

Published in Great Britain by Henry Kimpton Publishers, London
PRINTED IN THE UNITED STATES OF AMERICA

Preface

The name-of-the game in the quest for quality in living today is effective decision making. Being aware of the influences and options and choices which will determine one's behavior and actions is a principle basic to education for health today. *POSITIVE HEALTH– DESIGNS FOR ACTION*, in its second edition, addresses these principles and choices. As in the previous edition, it focuses on the most pertinent personal health decisions facing young adults. It is a book based on principles and not a lot of trivia and "nitty-gritty" pieces of facts and information. In many aspects, it is a book of highly selective, generalized, conceptual ideas concerning health problems and their possible decisions. Many designs are suggested—what is positive and of value to you must be your decision! We have endeavored to present only the major problems in an objective, helpful manner. All possible situations have not been stressed or even identified; many points and discussions have been placed in a section at the end of each chapter, entitled "Problems for Your Consideration" for three reasons: (1) The problems enable readers to pursue and explore their individual interests, based on prior experiences, interests and information; they provide an extension of the subject matter discussed in each chapter which can be investigated as well as being considered in a context of personal valuing and decision making; (2) Researching a problem requires an individual to become familiar with the personnel and material resources on the campus and in the community; (3) Investigating a problem often requires the skills needed in making health choices and may involve the individual directly or indirectly in a behavior modification experience.

We have opted for no photographs in order to keep the publication expenses as low as possible. We also wish to stress our use of the pronoun "he" in a collective sense and not in a narrow, stereotypic

v

restrictive sense. The pronouns he and she have been used so they may reflect the greatest meaning and understanding, sans discrimination.

We wish to thank John Phillips, Ph.D., Director, Health Education Cooperative for the NY-Penn Area, for his research and assistance in the chapter, "Improving Environmental Health;" we also wish to thank Edward Wickland of Lea & Febiger who had faith in the future of this second edition, ten years after the initial publication of the book.

Mary K. Beyrer
Wesley P. Cushman
Robert Kaplan
Columbus, Ohio

Marian K. Solleder
Greensboro, North Carolina

Contents

47714 ρ **2** ⁰

1

Your Health– Choice or Chance?

Cheers! Here's to you! Han Skal Leve! On the special occasions when these toasts are offered and your friends seek to honor you, your health is often the subject of the toast. Have you ever stopped to consider *why*, when actually there are few things that we take more for granted than our health? As long as we have the strength and energy to do what we want to do, we go merrily along our way with little thought to our well-being, per se.

We are willing to take risks with our lives and our bodies daily and do so almost casually. "Living dangerously" may be a lifestyle for many of us—perhaps too many of us! But, you may say, everything we do or don't do may involve a risk of some kind, and you are so right. H. McMillan said that to be alive at all involves some risk!

To most of us, health is either "good" or "bad," and not just a series of risks. So, when we pause to consider, we recognize that *health* means many things to many people. To some people, health is primarily a matter of *chance*: "I may or may not catch the flu;" "I may or may not get poison ivy;" "I may or may not get gonorrhea;" "I may or may not die of lung cancer, regardless of how much or how little I smoke." "It's all a matter of chance, anyway, and I'm willing to risk it!" To other people, health is definitely a matter of *choice*: "I have a thorough check-up every year;" "I prefer to eat a hearty breakfast every morning;" "I make it a point to get a booster shot for tetanus every ten years." Many of our routines or "health habits" are the result of choices that we once consciously made and often repeated and that now have become automatic in our daily schedules.

1

Perhaps the real questions are: What are the choices, and what are their bases? Are there some intelligent risk-taking behaviors that can be developed? Can the right decisions counteract the casualness of sheer chance? What about *you?* Is *your* state of health primarily a matter of choice or do you play Russian roulette with your well-being?

"HEALTH"—RESOURCE AND RESPONSIBILITY

According to many textbooks, health is a specific condition, although in everyday language health may be simply "what makes you tick." Actually, some definitions have much to offer for our consideration. Most formal definitions of *health* imply that it (1) is a state, condition, and quality; (2) incorporates a functioning coordination of the physical, intellectual, emotional, social, and spiritual factors; (3) is a means to an end (for example, happy, satisfying, productive living) and not an end in itself; (4) varies in degree from one individual to another and from one hour/day to another; (5) may be described as *optimal* insofar as the ultimate in degree is concerned; and (6) is reflected in a wholesome attitude toward ourselves and society.

Definitions of health which incorporate the majority of these characteristics are:

> Health is optimal personal fitness for full, fruitful, creative living.[6]
> Health is a quality of life involving a dynamic interaction and interdependence among the individual's physical well-being, his mental and emotional reactions, and the social complex in which he exists.[11]
> Health is the expression of the extent to which the individual and the social body maintains in readiness the resources required to meet the exigencies of the future[2]

These characteristics and definitions imply that health as a *complete* state of physical, mental, and social well-being simply does *not* exist; however, the interdependence and interaction of these factors is obviously critical. They also imply that one's well-being exists *for* something (both self and others) and not simply for its own sake. Health is something to be used; it is a quality which should help us live as successfully and happily as possible now, as well as being as ready as possible for the future. A third implication is that an individual with a congenital or acquired disorder can have optimal health as well as anyone else since the term *optimal* in this sense means the best or most favorable within the given set of conditions or circumstances. Essentially, optimal health is a matter of keeping all the relevant factors in as high a degree of performance and balance as possible, enabling you to meet your responsibilities effectively. A fourth implication suggests that health is a positive and dynamic state, rather than a negative and static one.

Thus, your health is both a resource and a responsibility. It is a resource which gives you sufficient endurance and fitness for everyday living as well as for times of emergency. It is a responsibility which stipulates that your friends, your family, and your community all have a right to expect that you will maintain the highest possible state of well-being. The degree or hierarchy of importance which we place upon fulfilling our basic physical and psychological needs as well as how we attain our proposed personal goals form a complex "health value system." The extent to which this value system is put into *action* is reflected in the degree to which we accept health in a positive context and as both a resource *and* a responsibility.

STATUS AND LEVELS

As a nation, we seem to be accepting and applying these concepts to some extent. We have not been content to leave all matters of health to chance, but rather have developed definite, organized, public health programs to make possible an optimal state of health for those who will accept the responsibility. Consequently, as a nation we have the greatest life expectancy in our history. Today a three-year-old child can expect to live an average of seventy-one and one-half total years; these data can be further interpreted to mean approximately sixty-eight years for boys and seventy-five for girls of that age in the white population and sixty-one and sixty-nine years respectively for non-white boys and girls. Obviously, these figures partially reflect what the differences in the socio-economic status can mean to health and the life span. Nevertheless, our current longevity is due in part to our low rates of infant and maternal mortality and our low mortality rates from communicable diseases. Today, Americans die primarily from accidents and the noncommunicable diseases, chiefly diseases of the heart, cancer, and strokes. Because we are able to control many of the communicable diseases, these diseases now appear primarily in the *morbidity* (illness) rates rather than the *mortality* (death) rates and statistics. The great advances in medical practice, surgical procedures, and pharmaceutical skills as well as the availability of hospital care have also played major roles in helping us attain our current health status.

We could mention many more factors which have contributed to our present health status. The high standard of living in the United States has produced better housing and better nutrition as well as more effective methods of sanitation and environmental control for both the individual and the community. Our voluntary and official health organizations are extensive, as is the amount of scientific health information which is made available to the public through the various communications media. We would be remiss to omit mention of such negative trends as the increases in incidence of venereal diseases, avoidable accidents, obesity, dependence on hard drugs, and alcoholism.

We can also view public health status in another framework. Let us assume that health exists in four levels: mortality, serious morbidity, minor morbidity, and positive health.[9] The lowest level, *mortality*, is that level in which few diseases and disorders can be prevented, controlled, or even survived. Fortunately in the United States, we have advanced through and beyond this level. The second level, *serious morbidity*, represents the level in which prevention, control, and treatment of most conditions are fairly successful. Today many of our medical personnel still are functioning within this level as they search for the causes of cancer, accidents, and congenital disorders. At a third level, *minor morbidity*, the emphasis shifts to minor illnesses such as respiratory problems and digestive disorders, which cause inconvenience and economic loss. Finally, at the highest level is *positive health*—our goal of optimal well-being in a safe and pleasant environment.

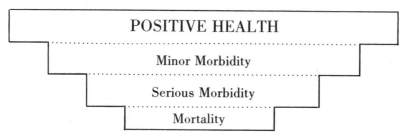

Fig. 1.   Four Levels of Public Health Status

Both the individual per se and individuals as members of a community must make intelligent choices based on the best scientific evidence, and then put them into *action* if we are to attain and maintain this positive health level for acquiring optimal rather than minimal well-being. Even today, too many of us are willing to settle for as little sleep or food or exercise as is necessary to "get by." Seemingly, our health just isn't that important until illness or injury "strike" and slow us down;

some people evidently do not put their health in a high value hierarchy. Most of us refuse to even try to live to our fullest capacity! The four greatest hazards to the health of the average American citizen may well be *fear, ignorance, apathy* and *quackery*. Perhaps the individual who is most likely to leave his well-being to chance is also most liable to fall into one of these four traps.

A major purpose of all health instruction is to *transmit* information that the research scientist has discerned to be basic to the maintenance of health. This is step one of a two-step process. This knowledge must then be *applied* and used by both individuals and communities. This is step two. Without the application the fact is useless! Of course, it is to be acknowledged that health facts will change as the researcher discloses new information; therefore, we cannot assume that our health practices of today will necessarily be those of tomorrow. However, the current gap between what we know and what we do is appalling. We have only to consider the thousands of needless deaths from cancer each year, deaths which could have been prevented if a physician had been consulted when the first symptoms appeared. Scientists have shown us how to *prevent* poliomyclitis and rheumatic fever, and how to wipe out tuberculosis. Our failure to use this knowledge is costly in both dollars and lives. Health instruction attempts to reinforce the fourth level of the health status levels, the level of *positive* health. But it is up to you to initiate the action that is necessary to acquire this level—you as an individual and you as a member of a community.

INTELLIGENT RISK-TAKING

It is quite evident that no one person or thing can *give* you physical, mental, and social well-being to help you "to live most and to serve best,"[12] Heredity already has partly determined your state of health. The physical and social pressures exerted by your environment are constantly influencing you. The values and beliefs evidenced in your home by such specifics as eating patterns, discipline theories, and recreation habits have played a role in forming your health behavior patterns. In addition you have been molded by cultural and subcultural elements including religion, race, and peer group relationships. The environment in which you grew up, whether it was in a rural or urban setting in the north, south, east, or west, has exerted pressure. The lifestyle which you are currently evidencing reflects your acceptance or/and rejection of many of these influences. Upon what bases are you making these decisions?

Life is a continuous do-it-yourself, problem-solving, decision-making process. The adequacy and effectiveness of your health is dependent upon your awareness of your needs, your weaknesses, your strengths, your values, your attitudes, and your self. Equal in importance is the knowledge that helps you determine when you can handle your health problems on your own and when you require professional help. It would be difficult, indeed, to overemphasize the part played by the specific motivating factor which prompts you to make the choice or take the chance and the role performed by your attitudes or feelings about the action in question. We are so easily motivated by attitudes and emotions; often scientific facts and principles are not the primary generators of our behaviors. Too often misconceptions, superstitions or "mood modifiers" are the basis of our decision. And this is one type of risk behavior that may be dangerous!

It has been intimated earlier in this chapter that taking risks does play a persuasive role in our lives. Godfrey Hochbaum suggests that "risk-taking" means a more or less thoughtful consideration of the probability that if you choose to act a certain way, a certain result will occur. You may arrive at the decision either through some actual deliberation or on the spur of the moment or in any other manner. Regardless of how you decide, especially pertinent is the fact that it is your *perception* of the risk and not the actual risk itself that is the crucial element in risk-taking behavior.[4] The greater the odds that you won't get the disease or the more uncertain the facts about the possible injury or the greater the psychological impact of your own belief or desire—all these play a far greater role in your decision than "deliberate, rational and conscious" consideration of the relative risks or probabilities. The way you feel rather than what you know is often what triggers the action.

Obviously not all risks are highly undesirable—or necessarily unhealthy or crippling—or imminently dangerous! There are many varieties, i.e., asking for a date for the first time with a particular person, or crossing the street in the crosswalk in fairly heavy traffic, or being in large crowds during a real epidemic of influenza.

The point is—we all take risks and chances as far as our physical, our mental, our social and our emotional well-being is concerned. We would like to assist you in taking those risks based on deliberate, thoughtful "scientific" considerations and value judgments rather than the spur of moment, haphazard whims or "gut" feelings or fears. The 1980's will be loaded with risks, many of which can be intelligently controlled.

One of the basic purposes of this textbook is to acquaint you with certain basic scientific principles, concepts, and guidelines regarding your health and to guide you to additional authoritative sources of information so that you may apply them as designs for action to solve your health problems. Such problems may include how to handle your tensions effectively, how to approach marriage and parenthood realistically, how to begin to protect yourself now against heart disease and cancer, how to cope with environmental health problems, and how to be an intelligent health consumer. Positive, optimal health is reflected in wise choices (and risks) to solve such problems. These choices, in turn, reflect the application of scientific principles coupled with an honest appraisal and awareness of problems as well as the recognition of the tremendous impact of your attitudes, desires, and values.

Positive health is a matter of sound, accurate *choices!* Positive health reflects a sound, effective design for action!

PROBLEMS FOR YOUR CONSIDERATION

1. When does risk-taking in health matters become sensible? Valuable? Stupid? Dangerous?

2. The modification of many of our health behaviors is dependent upon many different factors related to our value system. Specify and discuss the implications of several of these factors.

3. Identify and discuss some specific examples in which gaps exist between medical research or/and scientific information and health behavior.

4. Verify and discuss some of the current personal and national health problems whose solutions are obscured due to quackery, apathy, fear and ignorance.

5. Why is education for health considered by many to be a behavioral science?

REFERENCES

1. Dubos, René: *Man Adapting.* New Haven, Yale University Press, 1965.
2. _____: *The Torch of Life.* New York, Trident Press, Simon and Schuster, Inc., 1962, p. 11.
3. Gardner, John W.: *Self-Renewal: The Individual and the Innovative Society.* New York, Harper and Row, 1963.
4. Hochbaum, Godfrey M.: Cigarette Smoking: Is It Russian Roulette? *TRDA Bulletin,* 58:3, (March, 1972).

5. _____: *Health Behavior*. Belmont, California, Wadsworth Publishing Company, Inc., 1970.
6. Hoyman, Howard S.: Our Modern Concept of Health, *The Journal of School Health*, 32: (September, 1962).
7. _____: Rethinking An Ecologic System Model of Man's Health, Disease, Aging, Death. *The Journal of School Health*, 45: (November, 1975).
8. Michener, James A.: *The Quality of Life*. Greenwich, Conn., Fawcett Publications, Inc., 1970.
9. Report of the Chairman of the Technical Development Board to the Governing Council 1959-1960, *American Journal of Public Health*, 51:287, (February, 1961).
10. de Saint-Exupery, Antoine: *The Little Prince*. New York, Harcourt Brace and World, Inc., 1943.
11. School Health Education Study: *Health Education. A Conceptual Approach to Curriculum Design*. St. Paul, Minnesota Mining and Manufacturing Company, 1967, p. 10.
12. Williams, Jesse Feiring: *Personal Hygeine Applied*. Philadelphia, W. B. Saunders Co., 1950, p. 13.

2

Increasing Your Personal Effectiveness

The college environment today attempts to encourage the fullest possible development of the individual. It is an environment which fosters a desire for learning, reflective thinking, and social responsibility. Yet, unfortunately, a substantial number of the young people who start college do not finish. The reasons for drop-outs are many and varied, but the majority of students fail to receive their degrees because they lack personal effectiveness, that is, the ability to meet the demands of a changing environment.

When the student comes to college, he is given a measure of freedom that demands considerable maturity. In many instances he is just becoming independent of parental and other adult supervisors. In college he is asked to make a great many decisions for himself. He must organize his mode of life in a new environment in a way that is satisfying to him but in a manner that is acceptable to his peers and college authorities. He must also meet certain academic requirements to be "successful."

To be responsible for directing and controlling one's own life is no small order. It demands personal effectiveness. Personal effectiveness requires certain skills and competencies such as the ability to know oneself, to plan ahead, to control one's emotions, and to meet one's problems intelligently. This chapter is designed to assist you in developing a concept of personality in order that you may better understand yourself and others and to help you to develop plans for action to improve your effectiveness.

HOW PERSONALITY DEVELOPS

Your *personality* is the sum of your characteristics, and it develops through the learning process as you react to your environment. Both biological and environmental factors shape your personality. The old argument as to which is more important, heredity or environment, is fruitless. Nature and nurture play interdependent roles. Heredity is important, but we know that most genetic dispositions can be altered by environment. For example, a boy may inherit a physique potential of 6 feet, 200 pounds, but perhaps disease, an accident, or malnutrition keeps him from attaining this physique. Biological factors related to heredity affect adjustment and personality indirectly. Studies show that in junior high school the bigger and stronger youngsters hold more class offices and have greater status than their smaller and weaker peers. These large youngsters also develop different ways of adjusting in comparison with their smaller classmates, who often are smaller only because heredity determined that they mature physiologically more slowly than their peers. Heredity is also a factor in certain health conditions and is considered in the chapter on marriage.

After birth, the social environment begins to influence the child's personality. The individual is born with physiological drives and possibly, to a limited extent, with some psychological strivings. These compel him to satisfy personal needs. His social environment requires that he satisfy these in acceptable ways.

All people have the same general basic needs, which can be roughly classified as physiological, social, and self. *Physiological needs* are hunger, thirst, sex, activity, and rest. *Social* and *self needs* include a sense of belonging, feelings of affection, feelings of being wanted, and a desire for respect and success. Throughout life the individual strives to meet these needs. How he meets them is conditioned by factors in his environment such as the values and customs of his parents and companions, the laws of the land, the taboos of society, and the teachings of his school and church. If he matures in such a way that he has self-confidence and self-control, and in so doing develops behavior patterns that are reasonably satisfactory to himself and to his society, he is considered well adjusted. This does not mean that to be adjusted he must conform. Socialization permits a considerable amount of individual variation as does the uniqueness of the individual.

If the individual is able to meet adequately his basic personality needs, a motivating force involving a tendency toward positive growth called *self-actualization* may function. This force of higher needs makes possible the most advanced forms of thinking and aesthetic appreciation. Self-actualization brings to mind such words and phrases as independent and reflective thinking, perseverance, highly developed sense of values, creativity, scholarship and altruism.*

DIRECTING BEHAVIOR

Basic patterns of the eventual adult personality are acquired early in life. The *unconscious* mind plays an important role in directing behavior. Authorities in personality development point out that experience related to infant feedings, toilet training, and sex training, no longer remembered by adults, may be strong forces in determining how these adults may react to certain situations. For example, the helpless baby's life centers about getting food. He cries when he is hungry. If his mother comes and feeds him, he learns that crying is an effective way of relieving his hunger tensions. If he gets no response, he learns that there is no way to relieve a painful situation. Though this example is somewhat simplified, such early experience could lay the foundation for developing the attitude of either trying to do something about a problem or merely being apathetic about it. Drives and responses that are suppressed in early childhood and youth and cannot be talked about may be unconscious throughout life. (This may be due to the child's inability to communicate or because discussion of such drives is not permitted or encouraged by his parents.)

An infant can only demand and receive, but as he grows and develops, he learns that he must consider others. His parents and others discipline him by spanking, scolding, and explaining. Thus, he gradually develops a *conscience*. Conscience is a significant part of personality and is directly related to feelings of guilt. It can be described as a cluster of values socially acquired that tend to control bad behavior. These values are usually developed in early years and are acquired informally.[11] The conscience serves as a governor and directs the mode of expression of basic urges and drives. To avoid punishment or gain reward, the child behaves according to the rules of those about him. At first, the pressures to behave in certain ways are forced upon him. They are external. As he grows and reacts he makes them part of himself. As he begins to see himself as an individual, the external pressures give way to become values for self-guidance based on preference and

*For discussions of various personality theories see references 4 and 11.

self-respect. The mature person uses his conscience rather than fear to direct his behavior.

Conscious mental activity is voluntary and can be controlled. In adjusting to environment a person can be *self-directing*. He is superior to animals because of his higher mental processes: memory, intelligence, imagination, and judgment. He can call on these mental assets in choosing a course of action. Unfortunately, many of us never develop the skills for planning ahead and problem solving. We muddle through without using the information the sciences have given us. We never learn how to apply the scientific method to daily living. Designs for improving our conscious behavior will be discussed in the last half of this chapter.

Mental Mechanisms

Without defining or identifying them, we have discussed the so-called mental mechanisms of introjection, identification, and sublimation. These mechanisms are related to our growth process. *Introjection* is the process of absorbing the attitudes and ideals of those about us. Conscience partially develops this way. Most of our values and beliefs we have gained automatically from our parents. *Identification* is a mental mechanism known to most people as "hero worship." The boy imitates his favorite athlete, the girl her favorite actress, or vice-versa. As they develop, children unconsciously imitate their parents as well as absorb their values. Two health habits which are strongly associated with this process are smoking and drinking. Young people tend to follow the pattern of their parents in the use of tobacco and alcohol. *Sublimation* is the channeling of basic drives into socially approved ways of behavior. One learns to accept approved substitute goals for sexual or other drives that are blocked. A woman who does not marry early in life may go into a profession such as pediatrics or teaching where she can express love for people, especially children, in a constructive manner.

There are other mental mechanisms that we have blindly learned to use to reduce our tensions and solve our conflicts. Some of the most common of these are rationalization, projection, compensation, and conversion. *Rationalization* is a process in which we justify our ideas and behavior in a way that seems plausible to ourselves; for example, the young girl who has three examinations coming up on Monday reasons (illogically) that she should accept an invitation to date on Saturday evening with her boy friend as the date will prepare her for more efficient study on Sunday. *Projection* involves blaming our failures on others; for example, the athlete who feels his poor grade is because his professor doesn't like football players. In *compensation*, we make up for some real or imaginary inadequacy by doing well in another activity; for example, the honor student who substitutes outstanding grades for his lack of athletic ability. In *conversion*, we transfer the energy of a desire we cannot express into a physical symptom; for example, the student who comes into the college health service with complaints and symptoms of diarrhea resulting, unknown to him, from anxieties about final examinations. We use these mechanisms unconsciously to defend ourselves against anxiety, self-devaluation, and emotional hurt. To use these to some degree is normal, but overdependence on defense mechanisms is dangerous.

Adaptive Responses

One's personality is evaluated according to how he reacts to situations. One can handle problems by *flight*, *fight*, or *compromise*. These adaptive responses are sound methods of adjusting as long as they are used to solve problems realistically. The student who finds he cannot succeed in architecture may withdraw (flight) from that area of study to pursue another. Withdrawal, in this case, comes as a result of conscious direction. Students who dodge responsibility by faking illness or excuse-making are not responding in a healthful manner. The student who is doing poorly in a required course may use the fight reaction in a constructive manner by adopting the attitude "I can lick this one" and work harder to make a respectable grade, or he may use it in a destructive way by arguing that this requirement is absurd and the faculty doesn't know what it's doing. Early childhood experiences may well determine whether or not the fight and flight reactions are expressed in desirable or undesirable ways.

In *compromise* one does not attack nor entirely withdraw; he changes what he can in himself and the situation to solve his problem. The college sophomore gives up the idea of buying a sports car with money he earned during the summer when he realizes such an expenditure would require him to work during the school year. A job would take a great deal of his study time. He realizes that good grades throughout college may mean the difference between being placed in a highly desirable job or a less desirable one. He gives up the temporary pleasure and peer status the car would give him for a more important future goal. One learns to weigh the results, to accept what will be best in the long run.[4]

Mental Illness

As we noted previously, personality develops through learning, and many of our learned reactions and behavior patterns develop during early childhood and adolescence and may govern us unconsciously. If these patterns are reasonably satisfactory to both the individual and the social group to which he belongs and the individual feels good about himself, he is well adjusted. However, this is not always the case. In growing up, people sometimes develop ways of behavior that are extreme or inappropriate to the situation. If such behavior persists and interferes to the degree that one does not function effectively in his daily living, he is mentally ill. Perhaps the difference between the normal and the neurotic person is the extent of conflict with which he has to struggle. Or perhaps some people, because of their greater problem-solving ability, can better resolve their tensions. Then again, some people may be more subject to conflicts because of strong innate drives.

Compared with the behavior of the mentally healthy person, the behavior of the emotionally disturbed or neurotic person is different more in degree than in kind. Anyone may become afraid of deep water under certain circumstances, but some individuals, without knowing why, have a persistent and excessive fear of water. One would expect to have a feeling of weakness (*asthenia*) if he were unexpectedly asked to report to the office of the Dean. But some people have persistent and excessive weakness throughout the day for no obvious reason (*neurasthenia*). One expects to feel elated or depressed at various times and in various situations, but a few people have periodic attacks of melancholia or elation so marked that they cannot function with any degree of effectiveness in their daily living (manic-depressive psychosis).

Psychopathic (anti-social) personalities are individuals who apparently grow up in a social cultural background without the affectionate relationship of adults. They are without conscience and so have no sense of guilt. They know right from wrong but do not care. There is considerable range in this group from neurotic nuisances to criminals. They may have charm and poise which they use to manipulate people to gratify their own personality needs. Not all anti-social persons are psychopathic. They may have learned such behavior from their social environment.

The mental disorders just discussed have their origin in faulty personality development and are classified as neuroses or psychoses. The neurotic person usually does not need hospital care, but his effectiveness is impaired and he does need counseling to avoid severe personality difficulties. Psychoses are more severe than neuroses and the psychotic person usually requires institutional care. He withdraws, loses touch with reality, may show personality disorganization such as overexcitement and marked depression, or may have delusions of grandeur or persecution. The causes of the neuroses and psychoses are not known. Development is complex and not specific. In the case of psychoses there may be inherited tendencies which lower resistance to stress.

Some mental illnesses have a physical basis. The cause can be determined. Such illnesses are termed symptomatic as the disturbance is a sign of an organic disease such as a brain tumor, tertiary syphilis, or arteriosclerosis. Mental disturbances may also be produced by an overexposure to chemicals or drugs. Many of these mental disorders with known causes can be prevented or cured by established techniques.*

DESIGNS FOR IMPROVING PERSONAL EFFECTIVENESS

After giving some thought to this brief discussion of how personality develops, you may have concluded that at your age there is little hope for you to change your basic personality. You are partially correct. Even if you could appraise yourself quite objectively, intellectual knowledge of human development does not provide principles that you can apply to alter your unconscious patterns of behavior. However, conscious learning continues at any age and within the last two decades much has been learned which enables people to modify their behavior in specific situations and establishing better self-direction. College experiences provide you with opportunities to improve your self-image, your feelings of self-esteem. You can develop academic and social skills and competencies that will help you gain social approval. You can become knowledgeable about certain principles which, if conscientiously practiced, can improve your effectiveness in handling your daily living problems.

Apply the Scientific Approach to Daily Living

The scientific approach, as we have mentioned before, refers to the method of gathering and examining facts and using them to reach the best possible conclusion. At the same time, one realizes that new facts may necessitate changes in decisions and plans of action.

*For a more detailed discussion of mental illness see reference 11, Chapter 6.

It is not easy to apply this approach to your daily living as it requires objectivity, and in many situations you may feel insecure or threatened and seek to protect yourself. Yet, it is important for us to learn to use this approach as conflicts are part of living, and the way we handle them is important to our emotional and social life. You might begin to practice this approach by gathering facts on these questions about yourself.

How can I improve myself? The first step to improving one's self is to identify the self-defeating behavior you wish to eliminate and the desirable behavior you wish to increase. Some problems of college students are: Can I stop smoking? How can I lose weight? Can I get better grades? How can I be more attractive to the opposite sex? Why do I get angry so easily? How can I increase my time for reading? Why can't I be more pleasant to others? Many of these problems you can solve for yourself. The know-how is available. One method which you may be interested in learning about is behavior modification. This technique applies the psychological principles of learning to human problems and though it has definite limitations, the technique has been successful in dealing with specific problems such as those listed above.[16] (The reference just cited is used as a textbook in certain college psychology courses though Watson and Tharp feel the techniques for self-improvement can be mastered by the reader himself.)

Some popular books written by well-educated clinical psychologists, counselors, and psychiatrists have appeared on the market proposing theories for dealing with common emotional problems.[6,8] The authors of the references noted use clinical cases to substantiate their theories and have chapters telling when to seek professional care. Whether or not a reader can apply these without some professional help is not backed up by hard research. Since it is difficult for the lay person to judge the value of many such readings, the college student would do well to discuss such publications with professionals on the campus.

Are my goals realistic? Keep your goals high. Most individuals tend to underrate themselves, and some exaggerate their shortcomings to the degree that they feel inferior. Goals also can be unattainable. If, for example, you plan to be a doctor, you must be of high intelligence and able to maintain an "A" or high "B" average in college. If aptitude and psychological tests and past academic grades show little likelihood of such high performance, you may rightly conclude that your goal of becoming a physician is unrealistic. No one should change his aims on the basis of a score on a single test, but if a series of predictors contraindicate success in achieving a goal, you would do well to reconsider your plans for the future. Analyzing yourself in relation to goals is difficult. If you have doubts, you should seek professional help from the appropriate counselor.

Do I face reality? You must learn to accept what you cannot change or control. The college girl who thinks she can change her fiancé after marriage will be disturbed when she realizes this usually cannot be done to any significant extent. The driver who kills a child through no fault of his own may develop a deep-seated emotional problem unless he carefully thinks through the situation and recognizes that such things can happen—even to him. Do you realize that fear, anger, sex drives, frustrations, stress, and guilt feelings are normal and that it is how you function with them that should be your concern?

When do I need help with a problem? If you have difficulty in college without understanding why, you should seek competent help from the appropriate authority or agency. Many students can avoid academic difficulties if they seek help from a college advisor rather than some classmate, fraternity brother, or sorority sister. One needs competent help if he questions whether or not college is worthwhile, if his grades are not what they should be even though he is studying, if he is missing a lot of classes or examinations because of vague physical complaints, if he is always at odds with his instructors or people of authority, if he is depressed most of the time, and if he loses interest in others and tends to withdraw. Colleges have advisors for personal problems as well as curriculum and medical matters. The large university may provide special marriage, legal, financial, occupational, and psychiatric counseling as well. All of us need help from time to time. Do not hesitate to seek competent help when necessary.

Face Group Pressures Intelligently

The college population is made up of many small groups that have different values and so make different demands upon their members. Fraternities, sororities, science clubs, church groups, sports clubs, political groups: many colleges and universities have them all and you, the college student, face the problem "Will I join?" This may be a difficult question to solve as some groups appear to be more glamorous than others and obtaining information about what they stand for and demand is not always easy to come by.

It is well to remember that you join such groups to satisfy your basic needs for a sense of belonging, affection, satisfaction, and self-esteem. Therefore, it is important that you ask yourself such questions as: Are the demands of this group in conflict with my own convictions and values? What does belonging require in terms of money and time? Will belonging to this group help me achieve what I hope to achieve from my college education?

Joining certain groups and just attending college demand a certain amount of conformity. One conforms because he may be bombarded by propaganda to convince him that the goals of a group are valid, because he will meet with social disapproval, or because he may suffer certain penalties if he breaks the codes of rules and regulations.[4] You should raise these questions: Are they giving me a "snow" job? Will I feel at ease behaving as the group expects me to? Do the group's rules meet my standard of conduct? Does joining help me do anything more effectively?

Conformity is neither good nor bad. It serves the basic need of the group for self-maintenance, but blind conformity means giving up self-direction. Get the facts; don't let the "let's go along" attitude mislead you. The mature individual thinks for himself.

Develop Intellectual Skills

To improve mental efficiency, you should know that mental work follows the same law of function as does physiological work. You know that to develop a high level of swimming ability, you must swim. The same holds for intellectual skills. If you want to learn how to write, you must write. You might get a good grade by copying another student's term paper, but all you learn is how to copy. Learning comes through your own efforts. All the professor can do is guide your experience.

Many students do poorly in their academic work because they have not learned how to use their time well. They do not plan a regular study routine. Take out your class schedule and reproduce it on a larger scale. Put your courses on in red pencil—for your best effort your schedule must be built around your studies. Fill in other fixed times such as employment, meals, band, and sports. What you have left must be used for study, play, and rest. Set up your day time study hours carefully. Study after your classes by revising your notes in relation to the past assignment. Work out your schedule so you know what to study when. Your schedule is only a guide, but if used wisely it can improve your efficiency and give you more time. Your schedule must be flexible enough to allow for change but when tough assignments are made, borrow your time from study hours with light assignments. Do not steal time.

Inability to concentrate is the most common study complaint.

Physical or psychological distractions may be to blame. Studies show that noise interferes with higher mental task output. Even music can adversely affect study which requires critical thinking, though routine thinking may not be disturbed. In any case, if your room is noisy and interruptions by others frequent, it is wise to study elsewhere. The psychological factors that serve as distractors to concentration are related to anxieties—worries about grades, the girl friend, or conditions at home. If such psychological distractions persist so that they continually interfere with effective study, the help of a counselor should be sought.

The best learning experiences often occur when you study the material to be covered before going to class. If it is a lecture class, generally your instructor is going to cover material in your reading only to make sure that you understand it and can apply it or he will add new material to up-date readings. If it's a laboratory section, be sure to review the principles that are being applied. By studying before class you are in a good position to do two things: (1) ask intelligent questions to learn if you have the depth of understanding required; and (2) listen, since you need only take notes on what is not in your readings.

Taking examinations is a college necessity and even after twelve years of public schooling many students lack the know-how of approaching them. If you have good study habits, you have little to fear; but knowing something about tests and testing can help every student.

Find out what kind of test your instructor is going to use. If he plans to use objective questions, he will measure at the recognition and recall level of depth. If he is using essay type questions, be prepared for discussion and critical evaluation questions at a level of application and understanding. In taking objective tests, detail becomes important. Answer the questions you know and don't change these answers. Go back and answer those you're not sure of after you have been through the total test once. Find out how he grades them. If the test is long and hard to answer in the time he gives, he may use a right-from-wrong method of scoring. In taking essay examinations be sure you read the question carefully so you answer the question as it is stated. Organize it well and supply facts and evidence using illustrations when necessary to show understanding.

The authors of *A Time To Learn*[1] believe that self knowledge and knowledge of your environment are important to learning. Knowing such things as when you work best, and under what conditions you best concentrate are important considerations. They believe one can approach work in a positive manner rather than avoiding studying; you can learn "study behavior" if you realize personal change is possible and how to go about making those changes. *A Time To Learn* uses some behavior modification techniques mentioned previously.

Don't let poor grades get you down—find out the reason why you get them and do something about it.

React, but React Favorably

Emotions are normal and help us adjust.* Our feelings and moods are merely differing degrees of emotions such as fear, anger and guilt. They indicate how you are reacting to your social and physical environment. You need to learn how to control them. Control of such basic feelings can be accomplished through conscious effort.[15]

Fear is a basic emotion that is common to humans. Everyone has anxieties over finances, health, family life, and his own personal adequacy from time to time. *Worry* has been described as inefficient thought whirling about a pivot of fear. Even mild anxieties definitely hamper one's ability to think clearly. Every student has experienced poor results on an examination because he was so anxious about his grade that he could not concentrate on the test. Fear also impairs memory and perception. It affects people physically. It increases the heart and pulse rate, produces a dryness in the mouth, increases perspiration, and causes one to feel chilled and weak in the knees. Stress with anxieties over a period of time is the cause or a contributing factor of certain *psychosomatic* (mind-body) diseases such as ulcers, hypertension, and colitis.

The best way to deal with fear is to act. If you have a problem causing you to worry, you should ask, "Is it my problem?" A lot of people worry about things outside of their control. If it is your problem, a second question might be, "Is it my problem now?" If not now, you should make a note on your calendar when action must be taken. For example, suppose you are having difficulty in English 101 and have a paper to turn in Friday. You might worry about it all through the week, and the anxiety would hamper your study of other subjects. Instead, you should make a note: "Write English theme Wednesday evening; rewrite Thursday a.m. 10-12." You should then do it as well as you can and forget it. There is nothing that builds self-confidence as well as being up to date and prepared.

A way of dealing with fears is to identify them and develop the skills to carry on despite them. Remember that all humans have fears. If you can do nothing else, talk them out with a friend, instructor, counselor, minister, or doctor. No one is a coward because he fears.

*For further discussion of emotions see reference 4, Chapter 14.

Anger is a perfectly normal reaction. It has been estimated that the average man gets angry about six times a week and the average woman three times weekly. Men are more apt to get upset by inanimate objects such as a faulty car battery or some event such as tardiness. Women get angry at other people more frequently than men. The neurotic person has many pet peeves over which he gets angry. The well-adjusted person usually does not get angry unless thwarted in some manner. The well-adjusted person can take a kidding without getting mad; the neurotic person gets irritable.

Even though anger is normal, its frequency can be reduced. Plans for action which can be helpful include recognizing hostility as a fact, identifying situations that cause anger, and developing ways of preventing it from becoming chronic. Avoid discussion of difficult problems when you are hungry or fatigued. A discussion with Dad about those low grades will go better in the early evening after a good dinner. Don't bottle up anger, but rather, talk out your difficulties with a friend or interested person. A socially accepted way of expressing daily aggressions is through physical exercises. Over a period of time, failure to express anger may produce the same psychosomatic diseases as we mentioned in our discussion of fear.

Guilt is a perfectly normal emotion. It is essential if we expect responsible behavior from individuals, since it leads a person to correct lies, mistakes, and wrong doings. You can deal with guilt feelings by recognizing them, taking steps to make amends, seeking forgiveness, and avoiding similar mistakes in the future. Self-direction carries with it the responsibility of recognizing and correcting one's errors.

Pathological guilt occurs when a person feels completely unworthy because of some insignificant act or devalues himself for no apparent reasons at all. Such a person should seek professional help. He will usually suffer severe depression with his guilt.

Grief is probably handled best by expressing your feelings of sorrow in constructive ways. There may be anger, hostility, depression, and disbelief. Kubler-Ross in her book, *On Death and Dying*, explains that people who face death go through certain coping mechanisms: denial, anger, depression, and acceptance. The family also goes through stages of adjustment similar to the dying member.[10]

Fortunately most grief reactions do not incapacitate one for any length of time. There is a period of depression, loss of sleep, and often crying. Usually the support of friends and loved ones is sufficient to help most people through such trying times. Of course, reactions of individuals vary depending not only on the nature of the person, but the meaning of the loss to him. If the person is in some way connected with the cause of death, guilt and depression may be so great that professional help may be needed.

Suicide must be included here because it is related to emotional states and not necessarily mental illness. It may happen to the young adult in instances of compulsive reaction and in the older person with depression associated with grief of the loss of a loved one, terminal illness, or incapability. Students who have suicidal tendencies usually say that they may kill themselves or give other warnings less discernible. The suicide-prone student is a loner, he isolates himself, he is outside normal activities yet he may be a fine student. Observable changes in behavior include sudden neglect of school work, decrease in ability to communicate, change in life style, depression with withdrawal, and delusions.[2] None of these are uniquely characteristic of the suicide-prone student but when coupled with isolation one should be suspicious. You should intervene and ask him if he is troubled. You won't plant suicide in his mind if it's not already there. Encourage him to talk about his situation. Refer him to proper college or community health service personnel. Help him to develop friends and encourage him to participate in extracurricular activities.

Relieve Tensions Through Recreation and Relaxation

Daily tensions are bound to build up in our fast moving, status-seeking society. Relief can be provided through recreation and relaxation. Recreation may take many forms and provides opportunities for expressing aggressions and creativeness. You should consider two factors in selecting your own form of recreation. First, you should be able to schedule the activity frequently throughout the week. Second, you should pick out an activity that involves skills different from your work. For example, a woman who has a standing or sitting job who receives orders or complaints from others might be wise to select a competitive, big muscle activity in which she can express her aggressions in a wholesome manner and improve her muscle tone and circulation. The girl who is dancing each day for a musical comedy might be wise to curl up with a good book or play a game of bridge. College provides you with many opportunities to learn leisure time activities that you can carry on throughout adult life.

Learn to relax, that is, learn what kinds of relaxation are best for you. Too many people feel guilty about loafing. Doing nothing at the right time for a few minutes each day will help you to tackle your work with enthusiasm. Some psychiatrists feel that muscle tension actually causes anxiety. It is possible with practice to learn to relax complete-ly.[12] Of course, adequate amounts of sleep and rest are essential in preventing tensions. Minor irritations become major conflicts to a tired person.

A large number of young people are turning to transcendental meditation (TM) to relax and rejuvenate the body and mind. This simple technique reduces oxygen intake, heart and metabolic rates, and blood lactate producing a physiological and biochemical state of "restful alertness."[3] Its advocates claim that those who practice it twice a day for twenty minutes discover inner energy, overcome stress, and develop heightened awareness.*

Recognize That Mental Health Is A Family Responsibility

If you have understood our discussion of introjection, identifica-tion, and sublimation, you now realize that the family is the institution which plays the greatest role in shaping personality. For the most part, parents determine whether or not the child makes mistakes without being overwhelmed by them, whether or not he is game to try new things, how he feels about the world around him, and how he feels about himself.

Parents may favorably shape the personality of their child if they will stand by him when he gets in trouble, show him by their actions that they love him, let him know what is expected of him, and be consistent in their punishment of him. They should strive to follow these suggestions which are agreed upon by most mental health authorities. Parents should answer the child's questions honestly but only to the extent that he can understand the answer. They can assist him to become independent, to grow at his own pace, and to gain self-confidence by showing pleasure when he does well. They can teach him to be honest and sincere; studies indicate that people who have these characteristics have many fewer anxieties than those who don't have them. The young person who learns to tell the truth doesn't have to remember what he said. Parents can help him to establish worth-while goals. Frequently youths who do not have good parental models and controls recognize this. They should consider and then follow the activities of the many wholesome adult models in society.

---

*TM and other forms of meditations are now being seriously researched by behavioral and medical scientists to learn more about their potential benefits.

If conscientiously applied, the above designs for action can do much to improve your personal effectiveness. Although by the time you are in college your basic personality is somewhat fixed, you can continue to consciously improve your self-direction. Your life must have purpose and often to achieve purpose you have to learn to pass up momentary pleasures. Some of you will make wealth your long range goal; others will choose power. But there is evidence to show that the most successful and happy people are those who have learned to satisfy their needs by earning the respect and gratitude of others.[13,14]

PROBLEMS FOR YOUR CONSIDERATION

1. Identify a behavior you might like to modify during your college years. How will you go about doing it?

2. One must learn to function with the feelings of guilt, anger and fear. How do *you* handle *your* emotions? How can you become more effective in directing them?

3. Under what circumstance might stress be a constructive force in our lives?

4. Investigate the campus and community resources available to assist in the solving of student problems.

5. Explore Dr. Hans Selye's concept "altruistic egotism" as a way of coping with stress.

REFERENCES

1. Brandt, Phillip L., Meara, Naomi M. and Schmidt, Lyle D.: *A Time to Learn: A Guide to Academic and Personal Effectiveness.* New York, Holt, Rinehart and Winston, Inc., 1974, p. 206.
2. Berg, Conald E.: A Plan for Preventing Suicide, *School Health Review,* 1: (September, 1970).
3. Bloomfield, Harold H., M.D., Cain, Michael P., Jaffe, Denis T., Kory, Robert B.: *TM, Discovering Inner Energy and Overcoming Stress.* New York, Bell Publishing Co., Inc., 1975, p. 75.
4. Coleman, James C.: *Psychology and Effective Behavior.* Chicago, Scott, Foresman and Company, 1969, p. 293.
5. Chiang, Hung-Min and Maslow, Abraham (Editors): *The Healthy Personality.* New York, Van Nostrand-Reinhold Company, 1969.
6. Ellis, Albert, Ph.D. and Harper, Robert A., Ph.D.: *A Guide to Rational Living.* 1974 Ed., North Hollywood, California, Wilshire Book Company, 1974.
7. Gilmore, John V.: *The Productive Personality.* San Francisco, Albion Publishing Company, 1974.

8. Harris, Thomas A., M.D.: *I'm OK–You're OK*. New York, Harper & Row Publishers, Inc., 1969.

9. Jacobson, Edmund: *You Must Relax*. 4th Ed., New York, McGraw-Hill Book Company, 1969.

10. Kubler-Ross, Elisabeth: *On Death and Dying*. New York, Macmillan Publishing Company, Inc., 1969.

11. Lazarus, Richard S.: *Patterns of Adjustment and Human Effectiveness*. New York, McGraw-Hill Book Company, 1969, p. 472.

12. Rathbone, Josephine L.: *Relaxation*. Philadelphia, Lea & Febiger, 1969.

13. Selye, Hans, M.D.: *Stress Without Distress*. Philadelphia, J.B. Lippincott Co., 1974.

14. _____: *The Stress of Life*. New York, McGraw-Hill Book Company, 1956.

15. Viscount, David S., M.D.: Free Yourself from the Oppression of Bad Moods, *Today's Health*, 52:25, (March, 1974).

16. Watson, David L. and Tharp, Roland G.: *Self-Directed Behavior: Self-Modification for Personal Adjustment*. Belmont, California, Wadsworth Publishing Company, Inc., 1972.

3

Appreciating Sexuality

Sexuality is only one part of a total relationship—whether marital or non-marital. While recognizing this truism, controversy abounds over whether nature (biology) or nurture (socialization) determines sexuality. In health, a proper balance of physiological factors and environmental influences is maintained whether it concerns sexuality, physical fitness, mental health, or other aspects. The balance is not likely an even one. We can only know by experience that for each aspect of health, including sexuality, and for each individual, the influence of nature and nurture varies over a considerable range.

To be male or female is to be of one or the other sex. To behave in a manner characteristic of one's sex is to be sexual. Sexuality is the state or quality of being sexual—the expression of one's sexual drive and interest in sexual matters. It is a significant part of our personalities (the sum total of our characteristics and affects). As such it plays a major role in our interpersonal relationships.

Sexual activity can be exhibited in a broad range of behavior. Solitary sexual activity—as in masturbation; genital play or intercourse between same sex partners—as in homosexuality; male-female-heterosexual-sexual expression; and group "sex" are some categories of the range of sexual behaviors. The specific types of activities in which humans engage is a much more extensive list.

To be considered as a most important aspect of human sexuality is the degree of emotional commitment accompanying the physically intimate sexual act. Again, there is a range from one in which there is no emotional commitment to the unwilling partner (rape) to one in which a couple is "bonded" in love, fidelity, and sexual satisfaction for both until death.

Now, we also recognize a widening range of relationships or associations among individuals, couples and groups—the alternate life styles from the ever single to group marriage. Unmarried cohabitation is a growing phenomenon attributed to a social climate in which there is a questioning of traditional religious and sexual standards; a substantial feminist movement; an increasing divorce rate; improved and more available contraceptive techniques and abortions; more tolerance for others' views; and, in colleges, less supervision of students' private lives.

The quality of sexual expression in our interpersonal relationships depends upon our motivations and in turn upon our personalities. With the abuse of drugs we may choose to alter our consciousness to create a "different reality"—perhaps to create a more respected or lovable person than we perceive ourselves to be. Sexual exploitation, promiscuous sexual behavior, and pre-occupation with sexual matters to the exclusion of other developmental activities and responsibilities may also reflect insecurities and unfulfilled psychological needs.

To enjoy a healthy sexual life is generally dependent upon enjoying good health. In turn, we enjoy good health when we understand how we function, what we need and how we can best meet those needs in order to "live best and serve most".

THE PHYSICAL ASPECTS OF SEX

The male and female sex organs both complement each other, as required for sexual union, and are in some respects similar. In the human embryo there is no sex differentiation until the timely secretion of hormones from the gonads (primitive ovaries or testes). If the embryo is programmed by its inherited genetic structure to be a male, appropriate androgenic hormones will be introduced and the primitive sex structures will develop accordingly. In the female, no hormones are introduced and the female organs begin to develop at about six weeks. For example, the gonads become ovaries rather than testes. The penis and clitoris, the prostate gland and the uterus, the scrotum and the labia originate from the same embryonic cells.

Beginning at puberty, male sex cells, sperm or spermatozoa, are produced by the testicles, as are the hormones which cause the development of male characteristics such as muscular hardness, deep voice, beard and body hair. At puberty in the female, the ovaries produce the female sex cells, eggs or ova, and the hormones which

cause the development of female characteristics such as broader hips
and a more curvaceous figure, breasts, softer skin and muscle, and a
slightly different distribution of body hair. It may be said that a girl
becomes a woman when the estrogenic hormones begin to function.

The Female

In the female, after the onset of puberty, the sex organs undergo a
continuous cycle in preparation for bearing a child. This menstrual
cycle is the only human function in which a loss of blood is a sign of
health rather than illness. For most women, problems of the menstrual
cycle are non-existent or so mild as to require no alteration in normal
activity. For some, such difficulties as dysmenorrhea, painful menstruation, or amenorrhea, absence or stoppage of menstruation, may require
medical attention to obtain relief. Under the control of the endocrine
system, each month—or an approximation thereof—one ovary produces
an ovum which travels through the fallopian tube toward the uterus.
Ovulation, or the release of the ovum, usually occurs in alternate
ovaries. Sometimes, perhaps simultaneously, more than one egg is
produced. This can lead to the birth of fraternal or dissimilar twins.
While the ovum is developing, the uterus is building up a lining of blood
and lymph with which to nourish the potential embryo when it arrives. If
the ovum has not been fertilized by a male sperm, it disintegrates and
the blood and lymph are discharged through the vagina as the menstrual
flow. The period of discharge is known as menstruation. The approximate periods of the menstrual cycle are: first to the fifth day, menstruation; fourteenth day, ovulation; twenty-eighth day, end of the cycle and
again the onset of menstruation. Since the ovum can be fertilized for
only a brief period (estimates vary from anytime up to a few hours after
ovulation to two days), the fertile period occurs approximately at the
middle of the cycle. However, the only certainty about menstrual cycles
is their uncertainty. The term "approximate" is to be emphasized
because of the wide variations between individual women in the
schedule of their cycles and of variations within an individual from time
to time.

Menarche is the term designating the onset of a girl's first menstruation. The age range varies widely from nine to sixteen years or so, but
the average falls between eleven to thirteen years old. Approximately
thirty to forty years later, the ovaries will reduce the production of
estrogens and ovulation and menstruation will cease. This is known as
menopause. Though she can no longer have children, sexual relations
can continue. Recent developments in hormone therapy enable endo-

crinologists to consider prescribing treatment which delays or deceler-
ates the degeneration of female organs and characteristics.

The Male

The male sex organs are outside of the abdominal cavity and thus
are more easily visualized. Their function is comparatively simpler than
that of the female. There is no counterpart to the female menstrual
cycle, and after the onset of puberty the male is, in general, continually
ready to perform his role in reproduction. The testicles or testes are
contained outside of the body in a sac called the scrotum, where they
maintain a temperature 1 or 2 degrees lower than body temperature.
Sperm are continually being produced—by the millions—in the canals
of the testes and stored in a larger tube called the epididymis. When
stored sperm become too numerous, they are released or ejaculated
through the vas deferens and the urinary canal or urethra. The seminal
vesicle and prostate gland add fluid to form semen. So-called "wet
dreams" or nocturnal emissions are those quite normal occasions during
sleep when excitement occurs and the male unconsciously releases
accumulated sperm. Self-stimulation of the genitals, or masturbation, is
not necessary for the release of stored sperm. Masturbation, which is
normally engaged in by men more than by women, does no physical
harm. However, the traditional attitudes have categorized it as morally
wrong. Thus, those who practice masturbation sometimes experience
feelings of guilt and psychological conflict which may adversely affect
their sexual adjustment. The modern point of view is less negative in its
attitude toward masturbation. Some authorities contend it is beneficial
for learning and developing healthy sexual response.

Sexual Response

In both male and female, sexual response to stimulation is a total
body response. The work of Masters and Johnson is now renowned for
delineating the characteristic responses and for identifying four phases:
excitement, plateau, orgasmic, and resolution.

Generally, in the excitement phase, vasocongestion—an increase in
supply of blood to tissues or organs, and myotonia—increased tension of
muscles, are two mechanisms of response. Erection of the nipples, the
penis, the clitoris, and the engorgement of the labia are begun. The
heart rate and blood pressure increase. A skin flush or temporary rash
appears on the breast and lower abdomen of the female. A sweating
phenomenon, lubricating the walls of the vagina, begins. Fantasy,

touching and body contact, and sexual play or foreplay can heighten sexual tension and purposely prepare for coitus or sexual intercourse.

During the plateau phase, vasocongestion and myotonia continue to increase. The outer vagina is engorged, the clitoris withdraws or is covered by the hood. In the male, the penis increases in circumference, the testes increase in size, a skin flush appears and heart and breathing rates increase. In the female, the uterus raises up and the vagina develops an "orgasmic platform" in the outer third as the inner portion "tents" or deepens presumably to retain a pool of semen when received from the male.

During the orgasmic phase earlier responses attain their most intense or peak levels. A total body response with a uniquely pleasurable sequence of muscular contractions characterizes the orgasm. The male ejaculates the semen and the female experiences rapid, pleasant muscular contractions of the vagina and uterus which may continue as multiple orgasms.

The resolution phase provides for the reduction of vasocongestion (detumescence) and the relaxation of myotonia. Heart and breathing rates soon return to normal. Except in some youthful males, a refractory period or recovery period of some definite but varying period of time is required before stimulation and excitement to orgasm can recur. In the female, however, resolution is slower and re-excitement can often take place almost immediately depending upon preferences.

It is well to remember that no two human beings are alike and their sexual responses as well as their preferences vary. Further, it is a myth that only when simultaneous orgasms occur are sexual expression and pleasure fully realized. This theory can lead to frustration and unhappiness. Certainly, it isn't necessary for procreation.

Human Reproduction

During sexual excitement the spongy tissues of the penis become engorged with blood, causing the organ to become rigid and hardened. The erection enables the penis, during intercourse or coitus, to enter the vagina so that the semen and its motile sperm (approximately 250 million of them) can be deposited by ejaculation in the vagina near the opening of the cervix—the lower portion of the uterus.

Sperm deposited in the vagina swim up into the uterus and on into the fallopian tubes if favorable conditions exist. Movement is accomplished by the whip-like action of the tails of the tadpole-shaped sperm. Fertilization occurs if an ovum or egg, moving along the tube toward the uterus, meets a sperm which can penetrate its outer wall.

The ovum travels primarily by the wave-like action of the cilia, or hairs, lining the walls of the tubes.

With the union of the sperm and the egg begins a process of cell division and the potential development of a new individual. At the time of conception hereditary traits are determined. As cell division within the ovum takes place, the uterus, which has been preparing itself for supporting an embryo by storing blood and lymph, accepts the implantation of the fertilized egg and pregnancy follows.

PREGNANCY AND CHILDBIRTH

Among the early signs of pregnancy or gestation are unusual irritability, cessation of menstruation, sensitive breasts, and nausea or morning sickness. Frequently, the pregnancy is well under way before some signs are observed. Since the cessation of menstruation may not be due to pregnancy, laboratory tests which identify certain hormonal changes are the most reliable indicators of pregnancy in the early stages. For example, a sample of urine is taken and injected into a test animal, such as a frog or rabbit. If certain hormones are present in the urine, changes in the animal's ovaries occur indicating the probability of pregnancy. Tests are being refined which chemically analyze the urine in a few hours and which promise high accuracy in early identification of pregnancy. Occasionally such tests have to be repeated.

The embryo grows rapidly and begins to develop a placental attachment to the uterine wall. Later in the pregnancy, the placenta and umbilical cord pass food from the mother to the fetus and return wastes. After three months, the embryo is called a fetus and this is its designation until birth. The uterus stretches to accommodate the rapidly growing fetus, causing some displacement of other organs. The external physical changes are more visible but are only temporary. In addition to cessation of menstruation and ovulation due to hormonal action, other chemical changes occur such as the preparation of the breasts for lactation.

Prenatal Care

During the pregnancy, which lasts approximately two hundred and seventy days, the mother should receive adequate prenatal care from a physician or obstetrician. She would do well to follow sound health practices including a wholesome diet, with vitamin supplements if prescribed by her doctor. Actually, her health practices in earlier years may be more important. After the determination of pregnancy and an examination by the physician, routine visits will be made every three to four weeks for the first seven months or so. Then visits will be made more frequently—every week or two—depending upon the physician and the course of the pregnancy.

The physician usually checks to see that proper weight and blood pressure are maintained. Periodically, he or she will analyze the blood and urine. He or she may recommend that the mother give up cigarette smoking, since evidence indicates that mothers who smoke tend to have premature babies. He or she will check on the position and size of the fetus and measure the pelvis to determine if a cesarean section delivery is indicated. He or she will also check the blood for the Rh factor. (These conditions are explained later in this chapter.) In addition, during this time, arrangements for fees and periodic or prepayment plans can be worked out to reduce financial burdens.

Under proper care, various complications formerly common in pregnancies are now usually well-controlled. For example, toxemia, a form of blood poisoning due to metabolic disturbances in the mother, usually occurs in women unattended during pregnancy. A mother might have heart disease or diabetes, which would require close medical supervision during pregnancy. The likelihood of premature babies, that is, those under five and one-half pounds at birth, and infant mortalities are reduced by prenatal care. While our infant mortality rate is low, prematurity is a major cause of infant deaths and is associated with various defects. (Other conditions which require medical attention are discussed later in the section on congenital defects.)

The Birth Process

The amazing growth and complex development which lead from a minute cell, invisible to the naked eye, to a normal size baby, approximately six to eight pounds in weight and eighteen to twenty-two inches in length, is a feat of nature even more miraculous than man's harnessing of atomic power or traveling to the moon.

The process of childbirth is also a phenomenon of infinite magnitude. At the end of full term, and sometimes earlier, a hormonal change triggers the muscular uterine wall to start contractions. Known as labor, the discomforting and somewhat painful contractions are more easily tolerated with proper prenatal care and exercise and a wholesome attitude toward childbirth. Some anesthetic may be used to reduce discomfort. Early indications that the first stage of labor is about to begin are the rupture of the "bag of waters"—the amniotic sac containing the fluid which protects the fetus—perhaps a discharge of mucus, and intermittent contractions. With the fetus normally in a head-down position at this stage, contractions at the upper end of the uterus start moving the baby toward the remarkably elastic vagina, the birth canal. When the cervix is sufficiently dilated to allow passage of the head of the fetus into the birth canal, the second stage of labor begins. This is the actual birth of the baby. This stage is complete when the baby has been expelled by the force of the uterine and abdominal contractions of the mother, frequently assisted by the physician or midwife. As soon as the baby is born, mucus is cleared from its respiratory tract, the umbilical cord is cut, and silver nitrate or penicillin eye drops are used to prevent gonorrheal blindness. The third and final stage of childbirth occurs within about a half hour when the placenta and amniotic sac are expelled from the uterus. This is called the "afterbirth." The normal and natural process of childbirth which has taken place for untold generations is now safer than at any other time in history.

Breech and Cesarean Births

Normally, babies pass through the birth canal and greet the outside world in a headfirst position. In about 3 % of all births, babies present themselves buttocks and feet first. These are called breech births. The possibility of early respiratory function during the birth process, among other reasons, increases the risk in breech position deliveries. However, when anticipated, and with special handling by a physician, most of these births are successful and cause no greater discomfort than normal births.

In some instances, the pelvic structure of the mother is too narrow, the fetus is too large, or the mother's health is such that a cesarean section is required. In this case, the baby is delivered through an incision made in the abdominal and uterine walls. The fetus is taken before it enters the birth canal. Women may have several cesarean sections with no difficulty. Though the dictum "Once a cesarean always a cesarean" is usually followed, a physician may, under certain conditions, recommend that a subsequent pregnancy terminate in a normal, vaginal delivery.

HEREDITY

Parents are often concerned about the hereditary characteristics which may be passed on to their progeny and the possibility of defects or mental retardation. The science of genetics is still comparatively young, though much is already known about the transmission of inheritable traits from generation to generation. Genetic counseling at the time of the premarital examination can be most helpful, particularly if the family keeps accurate health records and medical histories.

Recent research into the structure of chromosomes and the role of DNA (deoxyribonucleic acid) in the transfer of genetic material is helping us to understand the process of heredity.

Inheritable traits are carried by the chromosomes in the nucleus of each cell of our bodies. Within each of 46 chromosomes are the multitude of genes responsible for specific characteristics. In the sperm and the ovum, only half this number of chromosomes is present. Thus, when the two unite in fertilization, the normal number of 23 pairs of chromosomes is restored. The element of chance comes into play when a random assignment of chromosomes occurs during the development of the sperm and ova. (In the female, development of ova begins before birth and the eggs are stored in the ovaries; in the male, sperm development occurs after puberty.) Chance continues to have its effect in determining which sperm with its particular genetic "message" will unite with which ovum and its particular genetic potential.

The sex of a child is determined by chance. The male produces two types of sex determining chromosomes, called X and Y. The female produces only an X type. Thus, an ovum can carry only an X sex chromosome, while a sperm may carry either an X or a Y sex chromosome. If a sperm containing a Y chromosome fertilizes the X-carrying ovum, a boy is conceived. The boy then carries an XY pair of sex chromosomes. A female carries only the pair XX. Of course, chance would be somewhat reduced if for some reason the male produced one type of sperm cell which was "healthier" than the other or the ovum tended to "select" one type of sperm cell over the other.

Chance may be reduced to choice by the findings of Landrum B. Shettles, M.D. of the New York Fertility Foundation. The X-bearing sperm-gynosperm has a larger, rounder head (carrying more genetic material). The Y-bearing sperm-androsperm has a longer tail and is speedier. However, the gynosperm seems to be more durable so if ovulation is late, it may still be available after the androsperm is "expended." Further, an alkaline environment favors the Y sperm. An X sperm can tolerate a slightly acidic environment—frequently found in the vagina—better than the Y. Perhaps because of the androsperm's greater fragility, normal sperm contains more Y- than X-bearing sperms. This may also account for the higher ratio of males conceived but also spontaneously aborted.

To improve choice, Shettles recommends to favor conception of a male: intercourse at the time of ovulation; prior abstinence; an alkaline douche of water and baking soda; deep penetration at the time of ejaculation; and female orgasm during intercourse in order to stimulate alkaline secretions. To favor conception of a female: intercourse without female orgasm; shallow penetration at ejaculation; and, intercourse only two or three days before ovulation preceded by an acid douche of water and vinegar.

Multiple births, usually twins, may or may not be hereditary. It is suspected that some women inherit a tendency to produce more than one ovum at a time. Thus, it is possible to have dissimilar or fraternal twins. A fertilized egg which splits into two separate units as the initial cell division takes place produces identical twins—each receiving exactly the same genetic material. In addition to a genetic tendency in the mother, the father's genes also stimulate the development of identical twins.

Principles that lend some predictability to the chances of inheriting genes that are paired differ in their effects. One usually dominates the other and is called dominant; the other gene is called recessive. Thus, if each parent carries a gene for the dominant trait dark eyes and a recessive gene for light eyes, the chances are 1 in 4 that the two recessive genes will combine to produce a light-eyed child. A general rule, which supports the belief that first cousins should investigate their background thoroughly before marrying, is that hereditary defects are generally recessive while normal traits tend to be dominant. Thus, if there is a history of a specific defect in the families of both partners, the likelihood of transmitting it to offspring is greater. A predisposition to the mental disease schizophrenia is probably inherited through paired recessive genes. Of course, other factors must be operative before predispositions or tendencies become manifest. A predisposition to diabetes is also considered to be inherited through recessive genes. Knowing that diabetes exists in the family should alert one to take steps to avoid its development, if possible, or detect it early so that it might be better controlled. In addition to rare inheritable cancers, a tendency to acquire cancer may be inherited. More recent studies indicate that certain viruses and an inherited tendency are associated causes in both diabetes and cancer.

Congenital Defects

Your chances of having normal children are far greater than those of having abnormal children. Estimates indicate that about 7% of the children born have significant birth defects.[4] Actually, almost all of us have defects to some degree.

Congenital defects, or birth defects, are imperfections present at birth due to abnormal embryonic development. Some defects, however, such as those involving the skeletal structure, teeth, heart, and other internal organs may not be detected at birth and do not become apparent until later life. Many birth defects are correctable, especially if detected early.

Heredity, genetic disorders or mutations, infection, radiation illness, injury, malnutrition or abnormal nutrition, and drugs or toxic chemicals are among the known causes of birth defects. Since congenital means existing at and usually before birth, defects due to injury during the birth process may be included.

Frequently, combinations of hereditary and environmental factors are multiple causes of birth defects. Diabetes, schizophrenia, and cancer, mentioned earlier as inheritable, are examples of birth defects which usually appear later in life. An inherited disposition to one of these diseases influenced by certain environmental conditions may precipitate the disease. An example which has received attention far out of proportion to its importance and unduly worries parents is the "Rh disease."

The Rh factor is an inherited component of human blood which was discovered in the blood of the Rhesus monkey. Under certain conditions, this chemical factor can cause a disabling and fatal blood disease in the human newborn. This hemolytic disease known as erythroblastosis fetalis occurs in only a small percentage of births. The problem is similar to that which occurs when ABO blood types are mismatched in transfusions.

When the Rh factor is present in the blood, as it is in more than 85% of the population, a person is said to be Rh positive. In about 13% of all marriages, the wife is Rh negative and the husband is Rh positive. Only in this small group is there a possibility of encountering any difficulty and even then it can usually be corrected.

Several conditions must prevail in order to cause a "yellow baby"—jaundiced and anemic as a result of erythroblastosis fetalis. First, the unborn child must inherit the positive blood factor from its father. If the father is heterozygous—inheriting both factors from his parents—the baby may inherit his negative factor. Frequently, it inherits the mother's negative condition. Second, there must be a "leak" in the blood vessels of the placenta which allows the Rh positive blood of the fetus to mix with the mother's negative blood. Frequently, no leak occurs or the leak is too small to be of immediate significance. Then, the mother's blood system must (a) react to the presence of the Rh positive factor, (b) produce antibodies with which to fight the "foreign" Rh positive cells, (c) produce antibodies in dangerously large quantities, and (d) pass the antibodies through the placental membrane into the blood of the fetus.

In Rh-incompatible couples, less than 10% of all births are affected. Sensitivity and production of antibodies increase in mothers only if, in subsequent pregnancies, the fetus inherits the father's positive factor. Even if this allergy-like reaction (which is also similar to the development of immunity to infectious disease) develops, it is possible for the physician to control the disease.

A precautionary measure during prenatal care is to conduct periodic blood tests for the presence of antibodies in the mother's blood. Fortunately, this would occur late in the pregnancy. If severe enough, and it rarely is, the obstetrician may elect to induce early birth to remove the fetus from the now hostile environment. Also, he or she will be preparing to transfuse the blood of the newborn with compatible Rh-negative blood. The baby will produce Rh-positive blood which will restore itself in the system. A technique for transfusing blood when necessary into the unborn fetus is currently under development. In many ways, the Rh problem is more the concern of the physician than the parents.

While mental retardation, as well as other defects, can be caused by erythroblastosis fetalis, other diseases are more significant. Mongolism, for example, is the most common cause of mental retardation. This is due to a genetic disorder in which there is an extra chromosome or a translocated—misplaced—chromosome. This occurs in an estimated 1 to 1000 live births.

Infectious diseases are also a factor in birth defects. If the mother has the German measles (rubella) during the first three months of pregnancy, there is a 20 to 30% possibility of having a baby with a brain, hearing, vision, or heart defect. Syphilis can be transmitted from mother to fetus and defects result. Gonorrhea can cause blindness if, during the birth, the infectious organism in the vagina gets into the fetus's eyes and if appropriate eyedrops are not given.

The fact that many of these conditions are preventable or can be corrected demands greater attention. While the list of defects appears long, we must remember that most babies are born normal. In addition, there are many choices which can be made to reduce the chances of encountering serious congenital defects.

CONTRACEPTION

The essentials of reproduction are components of the healthy reproductive systems of the male and female: an ovum capable of being fertilized, active sperm capable of fertilizing an ovum, an unobstructed route for their passage, and a uterus favorably disposed to maintaining a developing embryo.

Sterility and Infertility

Either temporarily or permanently, in one or both partners, one or more of the essential components may not be met.[2] The terms sterility and infertility are used to designate this condition, though sterility is generally used to indicate a permanent condition.

Infertility can frequently be reversed. Blocked tubes, a malpositioned uterus, hormonal deficiency, inadequate quantity or quality of sperm, undescended testicles, and unfavorable emotional conditions are among the causes of infertility that are often correctable. These conditions are no reflection on one's masculinity or femininity. They may be inherited or acquired defects—perhaps due to measles, venereal diseases, or other diseases. Certainly, if children are desired, premarital examinations and postmarital counseling can be important aids to reducing infertility. However, if necessary, adoption can become a highly satisfactory alternative.

Miscarriage and Abortion

A nonliving embryo or fetus that becomes detached from the uterus prematurely (less than 28 weeks) and is expelled is said to have miscarried. Miscarriage or spontaneous abortion occurs about once in every 15 pregnancies and usually takes place in the first three months. Studies of miscarried embryos and fetuses have shown that a vast majority were defective or abnormal. Thus, a miscarriage may reasonably be considered a blessing in disguise. Chronic miscarriage may be related to the health status of the potential mother and requires medical attention.

Artificial or induced abortion is the elimination of the embryo by chemical or mechanical means. Chemicals and drugs are not too effective and are frequently injurious, even fatal, to the mother. Mechanically induced abortion, that is, with the use of instruments, requires competent medical procedures.

In a pregnancy of less than twelve weeks (from the first day of the last menstrual period), one of two abortion techniques may be used. The oldest is the D & C or *dilatation and curettage*. The cervix is opened—dilated—gradually by inserting wider and wider rods until the physician can use a forceps to remove fetal material and then to scrape the endometrium or walls of the uterus gently with a curette. A D & C takes about twenty minutes.

A new technique for a first trimester abortion is by vacuum aspiration. Though not always necessary, a local anesthetic at the cervix (paracervical block) is applied before inserting a cannula or curette attached to a suction instrument and therefore called a *vacurette*. Fetal material is drawn from the uterus rather than scraped or spooned from its walls. This method is faster and, in some respects, safer.

Later than twelve to fourteen weeks, usually not earlier than sixteen weeks, a procedure which may be used is a form of *intrauterine injection* known as "salting out." Some amniotic fluid (which surrounds the fetus) is removed through a long needle through the abdomen and is replaced by a strong salt solution. About twenty-four hours or so later, the woman will experience labor contractions and subsequently expel the fetal material as in a spontaneous abortion.

An older method, sometimes used in the second trimester, is the *hysterotomy*. This is a surgical procedure which means "to cut into the uterus." Usually this occurs through the abdominal wall but is sometimes approached through the vagina. Hospitalization is required as is a more extensive recovery period.

To improve on surgical methods of abortion there is the developing use of *prostaglandins*. This class of drugs was first found in the semen of man and sheep and can cause contractions of smooth muscle. Though not yet completely effective, intravenous administration of prostaglandin may become an important method of inducing abortion.

The legalization of abortion has had some social as well as individual benefits. Death rates due to abortion, and maternal and infant death rates, have been substantially reduced. Immature births, abandoned infants, out-of-wedlock infants, and low-birth-weight (high risk) babies have all been reduced.

While abortions are becoming safer—even less dangerous than giving birth—and more convenient and less expensive, they are not without hazards. Perforations of the uterus, bleeding, and infection can occur. Repeated abortions increase the risks. Of course the earlier in the pregnancy the abortion, the less the risk. Moreover, there are psychological-emotional considerations. Choosing from among types of abortion may be secondary to choosing from among alternatives of which abortion is only one. Counseling services associated with some agencies and abortion clinics can be helpful. They also provide an opportunity to consider contraception and sterilization.

Children can be blessings when wanted; when unwanted, they are felt to be burdens and may suffer from rejection. To permit a newly married couple to make adequate marital adjustments, the first pregnancy should be deferred for a year, possibly two. For health reasons it is preferable for mothers to have children no less than eighteen months or two years apart. Financial as well as health considerations help to determine child spacing and the number of children a family should have. Individual couples' choices will vary widely, however.

Family planning or *birth control* though less so now is still a controversial subject. While the Roman Catholic Church opposes mechanical and chemical methods of contraception, it does not oppose the more natural rhythm method. In any case, the method of family planning, whether by pill, device, or natural methods, is a matter of individual choice. Contrary to popular belief, such organizations as the Planned Parenthood Federation have not been primarily interested in preventing births. Their main interest has always been to help families plan their growth. Population control has become a factor in planning family growth.

If sexual intercourse is to be enjoyed, a couple—married or unmarried—should know about and use contraceptive techniques at the outset. Young women are known to become pregnant as a consequence of their first coitus. (On rare occasions, during heavy exposed petting and non-penetrating mutual masturbation, sperm deposited outside the vagina have succeeded in finding the ovum.)

Non-Prescription Methods

While "any method is better than no method at all," the methods in this grouping are easier to obtain. The first is really not so easy for some but needs mention, and those who select it need support and reinforcement. *Abstinence* is a way of life for some, but for most the restraint and self-discipline required to abstain from all sexual activity is too much.

Coitus interruptus, or withdrawal by the male before ejaculation, is the oldest and perhaps widest used natural method in the world. Unfortunately, the failure rate is quite high and many couples find it an unsatisfactory experience.

The *condom* or rubber sheath is an old, fairly reliable method of preventing sperm from entering the uterus. When properly worn on the erect penis, it serves to collect the semen. However, it does sometimes break or slip off, causing a spill of semen in the vagina. Condoms are also called prophylactics because they were originally used—and still are—to help prevent venereal disease.

Chemical-spermicidal methods include foams, creams, and jellies which can be purchased easily. Applied directly or through applicators, they are used to block the cervical opening and to immobilize and kill sperm. Used just before each sexual intercourse, they are reasonably effective. Combined with the male's use of a condom, the proper use of these chemicals can attain a high contraceptive success rate. Vaginal foaming tablets and vaginal suppositories are among those "better than nothing" products.

The Safe Period or Rhythm Method is not quite safe enough. But it is a method to be considered by those whose religious beliefs limit the alternatives. The method is based on the fact that pregnancy occurs around the time of ovulation; the difficulty is in predicting that time. As noted earlier, the menstrual cycle is uncertain and professional help may be needed to calculate the potentially safe days which may be too few to be satisfactory.

Douching is not a recommended method, since it is closest to "no method at all." Rinsing or syringing the vaginal canal after intercourse is usually too late to "wash out" sperm and may even encourage their dispersal toward the cervix.

Methods Requiring Medical Supervision

Among the methods requiring a physical examination and prescribed by a physician, probably the best known is "the pill." *Oral contraceptives* include many different birth control pills which generally fall into two classes, combined and sequential.

In each case, two synthetic hormones—estrogen and progesterone —are the essential steroids influencing hormonal birth control or *ovarian steroid contraception.* The combined or classical pill contains both hormones in each pill. In the sequential series, the first 15 or so pills are only of synthetic estrogen, while the last 5 are made of both synthetics. Though in small quantities, compared to the production of natural hormones, progestogen—the synthetic progesterone—is the main actor. Estrogens are used in smaller quantities. For those who cannot or will not tolerate the effects of estrogens, a new "mini-pill" of progestogen only can be used. It is not as good as the combined but almost as effective as the sequential pills.

The primary effect of the pill is to prevent ovulation. The additional hormones influence the system in such a manner as to represent pregnancy (without the fetus). For some women the temporary side effects are like those of early pregnancy.

Failures in the use of ovarian steroid contraception are mostly due to forgetfulness in taking a daily pill. Some schedules provide placebos, pills with no real effects for the "neutral" days before menstruation but to help maintain the pill-taking habit.

To make the process still more reliable (and thus convenient), long term injections and implantation of hormones are coming into use. A "morning after" pill is also under development though currently used in some extreme cases such as after a rape.

The safety of ovarian steroid contraception has been under serious study for some time. Its use has been associated with cancer, thrombo-embolism (blood clots), and several other conditions. When, with the physician's evaluations, women at risk are given other methods of contraception, complications are reduced often to less than those of undergoing a full-term pregnancy and childbirth. When fertility is desired, it can be restored usually within three months after discontinuing the use of the pill.

Intrauterine Devices

A method almost as effective as the pill and more convenient in many women, is the IUD or intrauterine device. Its effectiveness is rated at 1.5 to 3 pregnancies per 100 women-years (100 sexually active women of child-bearing age over the course of a year).

There are several types of IUD's, which must be inserted into the uterus by the physician. Once there, women generally need do nothing more than occasionally check for its continued presence. Made of plastic or nickle-chromium alloy, and some with copper, the most common are the Lippes Loop, Saf-T-Coil, Birnberg Bow, Dalkon Shield, and Copper-7.

Recently the Dalkon shield was withdrawn because of complications it was suspected of causing. The Food and Drug Administration has re-approved its use under continuous supervision by the physician. The Copper-7 is the IUD often used and recommended in Planned Parenthood Clinics.

Contraception by the IUD is believed to occur by causing a speed-up in the ova's movement through the fallopian tube, reaching the endometrium before it can receive it. That is, implantation cannot occur. Or perhaps its presence causes a chemical reaction in the endometrium that prevents implantation or even that interferes with the sperm's passage into the tubes. Since the actual method of effect is not known, many authorities consider IUD's to be abortificients (abortion-inducing agents).

Some women experience cramps for a while after insertion. Some women cannot retain an IUD; their uterus expels them, though re-insertions and different IUD's may lead to successful retention. Danger-ous side effects, such as uterine perforation and infection, are rare. Annoying cramps and bleeding or spotting occur but usually disappear in three or four cycles. Women who have not yet born a child (nullipara) may have more discomfort with an IUD than women who have (unipara or multipara). In any case, there are still alternatives.

The Diaphragm

To prevent sperm from traveling into the uterus, obstructive devices (the condom is one) have long been used. A modern relatively effective procedure is the use of a diaphragm. This is a dome-like or bowl-like thin rubber sheet molded onto a springy metal ring.

Diaphragms must be properly sized to the internal anatomy of the female. They can be inserted by fingers or with an applicator. To be effective, a spermicidal jelly is applied to the diaphragm, particularly around the ring or rim before insertion. Alone, the diaphragm is not an effective contraceptive.

Sometimes diaphragms slip out of place, are removed too soon (less than six hours after intercourse), are no longer properly sized, or even develop a puncture. Some users complain of the "bother" their use seems to cause. Nevertheless, this is a viable and relatively successful contraceptive for those who cannot use the pill or IUD and also do not want to risk other methods or find them less satisfactory.

The Cervical Cap

Like a smaller diaphragm, a small rubber cap fitted to the cervix can be worn for longer periods. Application is a bit more difficult for some women and a spermicidal jelly may or may not be used. Its advantage over the diaphragm is that it can be applied at a time separate from sexual intercourse and is considered less "disruptive."

This discussion of "prescribed" contraceptive methods, as well as those that are available without a physician, presents alternatives that are easily reversible when children are desired. Also, they seem primarily to be the responsibility of the female. Until newer methods effective for males are available, and as additional alternatives to unwanted pregnancy and children, there are surgical and more permanent methods to consider.

STERILIZATION

Vasectomy

A relatively minor surgical procedure, but highly significant to the individual, is done often in the physician's office (usually a urologist). A vasectomy is the cutting of the vas deferens of both testicles and then tying (ligation) or clipping the ends of this tube or cauterizing them by electrocoagulation. The incisions in the scrotum to expose the vas deferens are often so small as to sometimes be left without stitching. Local anesthesia is used and many men go on their way; others elect to rest and relax for a day or two.

After surgery, sexual intercourse requires use of a contraceptive until semen no longer contains sperm. At least ten ejaculations are required before sperm stored in the upper vas or ampulla are cleared out.

This method rarely fails except when the ends of the vas have somehow become reconnected or *recanalized* or perhaps the surgeon severed the wrong tube or there may have been a congenital duplication (two) of the vas on one or both sides. Sometimes there are discomforting side effects like bleeding as a consequence of surgery or an infection sometimes of the epididymis.

A vasectomy should not be considered reversible. Therefore, serious consideration should be given by the male and his partner or wife before choosing this permanent method. However, it is safe, effective, simple and short (requires less than a half-hour), inexpensive, and convenient. Males may need counseling to be assured that masculinity, hormone production, and sexual performance and desire (libido) are in no way impaired. This means only a healthy, well-adjusted male is the best candidate for this alternative.

Tubal Ligation

In the woman there are a few surgical procedures which cause permanent sterility even if the operation is performed for other reasons. Removal of the ovaries—*ovariectomy* or *oophorectomy*–is performed for other more serious conditions than voluntary sterilization. *Hysterectomy,* or removal of the uterus, is done only for some pathologic condition, and sterilization may be a secondary effect. The same is true for the removal of the fallopian tubes—*salpingectomy.*

For voluntary permanent sterilization in the healthy female, the method of choice is a tubal ligation or *laparotomy.* The fallopian tubes are cut, tied or clipped or cauterized to prevent the passage of ova to the uterus.

Often the operation is done shortly after childbirth while the woman is still in the hospital. An abdominal incision or an incision through the vaginal wall provides access to the tubes. Newer techniques have made the procedures more convenient and less discomforting. A laparoscope is inserted through a small abdominal incision to sight the tube; a second instrument through another small incision cauterizes and cuts the tube. A culdoscope is used for a vaginal approach and usually only a local anesthetic is necessary.

While there are a few failures, this is a permanent procedure. Rarely can there be an intentional reversal. Generally, a vasectomy is a better risk than a salpingectomy. The woman should be emotionally healthy and certain of her choice.

HAVING CHILDREN

To many of us, married or not, having children is an important part of life and happiness. Some couples cannot or do not choose to have children. This can be better than having unwanted children. For those who desire children but cannot have them naturally, there is always the alternative of adoption. Also, those with hereditary defects may wish to consider this alternative. With the population growth as a real concern, adoption is an excellent possibility.

Others of us can develop quite satisfactory relationships and lifestyles without children in our families. Some may derive satisfactions from a variety of sources while making a social contribution.

SEX AND LOVE

In our society, children generally represent the fruition of that profound relationship called love. Wives want to bear and raise children born of their love. Husbands want to father and be responsible for their wife's children. These are not children born of necessity—children required for economic or survival reasons—but the products of desire or choice. An intimate personal display of affection and respect is represented in the wholesome sexual relationship of love in marriage. Sensual satisfaction is important, but it is not the only reason for the sex act. The immature individual, the exploiter, and the domineering male of the past, who demanded sexual submission of his wife as a part of her "duty," have no place in modern marriage. Present knowledge of contraception and family planning enables married couples to express and enjoy their love in its deepest sense without fear of overburdening their families or "overpopulating the earth."

Many young couples do not realize beforehand that mutually satisfactory sexual adjustment in marriage frequently takes longer to attain than other areas of adjustment. This is not true for all couples, but unrealistic expectations of sex can make adjustment difficult. Mass media such as movies, magazines, television, and advertising misinform by giving the impression that mutual sexual satisfaction is easily attained. Perhaps on more primitive levels of expression, this would be true. However, even as an act of mutual love, some of the factors that can aggravate the complexity of making a good sexual adjustment are the man's relatively quick readiness for sex and the woman's slower developing readiness, and other factors such as fatigue, poor health, fear of unwanted pregnancy, and unsatisfactory premarital experience. Chastity before marriage, sometimes belittled, is still a widely held value. It is also considered an important foundation for the structure of our society. Violations of moral and religious codes frequently lead to guilt feelings and conflict which can adversely affect sexual adjustment. More enlightened attitudes toward the wholesomeness of the human body, the role of sex and the sex act, and the marital relationship have made the mutual satisfaction contributing to a happy marriage possible to ever-increasing numbers of people. To the extent that we have been properly oriented toward sex and its meaning by parents, church, and education, we can more readily achieve sexual adjustment in marriage or out.

THE PREMARITAL EXAMINATION

A significant aid to the reduction of problems and the attainment of adjustment in marriage is the *premarital examination*. In most states, the only requirement by law is a blood test of both partners before a marriage license is issued. If syphilis is found, the license is withheld until adequate treatment is obtained and further tests prove negative.[3] Too often, young couples believe that the blood test is an adequate premarital examination. One blood test does not constitute an examination. Many factors *enter into a health* appraisal.

At least several weeks—preferably a few months—before marriage the couple should be examined by a physician. Either or both partners may have had no medical checkup for several years, and to start a marriage with undetected and uncorrected defects or in poor general health would be a serious handicap. Diseases such as heart disease and diabetes which may contraindicate childbearing may be discovered. Rarely, but significantly, anatomic defects which may prohibit or affect childbearing and sexual adjustment are found. Blood typing, particularly with reference to the Rh factor, may be considered at the time of an examination. In such cases, correction and counsel by a physician is indicated. Intimate counseling with both partners on matters of sexual adjustment, fertility, hereditary characteristics, and state marriage laws may be necessary.

Making such decisions, which can properly and mutually be arrived at before the wedding, reduces the possibility of later difficulties. In the event that the rhythm method of contraception is to be practiced, the woman will want to see her family physician or gynecologist a few months before the wedding so that her menstrual cycle can be determined. Couples should remember that excitement such as preparation for the wedding and honeymoon may alter the cycle. Those who prefer may be given information concerning contraceptive pills or be fitted with contraceptive devices. For some women, the hymen, a membrane which partially blocks the opening of the vagina, may have to be stretched prior to sexual intercourse. Formerly, it was believed that an intact hymen was evidence of virginity. However, this membrane can be ruptured inadvertently in the course of normal activities.[3]

Too frequently, only the woman obtains premarital examinations and counseling services. The man normally has no superior education or background in these matters. He will do well to recognize his responsibilities. Though it may be preferable to visit his own family doctor for his personal examination, both partners should be present when being counseled on marital adjustment.

Not all physicians are adept at premarital counseling. Nor can they always anticipate your greatest concerns. You should be prepared to speak frankly and to ask the questions you want answered. Such matters as establishing a desirable frequency for sexual intercourse, expectations for orgasm or complete satisfaction (particularly for the woman), and sexual techniques are best discussed with the physician by both partners. Sexual adjustment in marriage can be one of the more difficult problems. For the most part, ignorance and misunderstanding contribute to it.

Clergymen, family life educators, and marriage counselors can be valuable in supplementing the counseling aspects of the premarital examination and discussions with parents. For some marriages, the value of recognizing the need for and obtaining the qualified, objective services of a counselor during marriage, as well as before, cannot be overestimated.

Love, sex, marriage, children, and health do not happen entirely by chance. Fatalistic attitudes or belief in predetermination are philosophical expressions of the helplessness of man and his submissiveness to chance. Our design for attaining and maintaining optimal health is aligned with enlightened self-determination, rational thinking, and the control of choice. Contrary to the abandonment of personal responsibility to "luck" in the lore of romance—which some segments of our culture tend to promote—successful, happy family life is largely a matter of *choice*.

PROBLEMS FOR YOUR CONSIDERATION

1. Women campaign for equality between the sexes. In what ways can equality be established? In what ways are the sexes similar and dissimilar?

2. What is gender identity and gender role? Identify examples of how they might differ. How are males and females conditioned or socialized for their appropriate sex behavior?

3. Masturbation is said to lead to a more intense response than sexual intercourse yet most prefer the latter. Why? Does masturbation influence sexuality in constructive or destructive ways?

4. What are some of the possible consequences of the use of drugs during pregnancy? Explain some of the most recent developments in the control of severe birth defects.

5. Several authors such as Kirkendall, Duval, Reiss, Hettlinger and others have written on values, morals, and standards of sexual behavior. Can you identify their main themes and the components of loving behavior? What is love?

6. Outline the important considerations of planning for marriage. Where do we need to provide parenting education and of what should it consist?

REFERENCES

1. Novak, Edmund R., Jones, G.S. and Jones, H.W.: *Gynecology.* Baltimore, The Williams & Wilkins Co., 1971, pp. 272-284.
2. Oliven, John F.: *Clinical Sexuality.* 3rd Ed., Philadelphia, J. B. Lippincott Co., 1974.
3. Trythall, Sylvester W.: The Premarital Law. *JAMA, 187:*900, 1964.
4. Volpe, Peter E.: *Human Heredity and Birth Defects.* New York, Bobbs Merrill Company, Inc., 1971.

4

Using Psychoactive Drugs

The trouble with drugs is people. There is no way we are going to eliminate drugs or to develop absolute control of their availability. After all, medicines are drugs used to prevent, treat, and cure disease and promote health. Pharmacologically, drugs are chemical substances which influence the structure and/or function of living organisms. Many different drugs are used to relieve pain and discomfort. Some are used to relieve psychological or emotional pain.

Mood-modifying or consciousness-altering or psychoactive drugs abound in nature and are synthesized by man. Some are used in their natural state like the coca leaf of South America where the Peruvian and other indians chew it for its mild stimulating effect. Some require a modest amount of processing like roasting beans and making coffee or curing tobacco. Marijuana can be used with little or no processing. Alcohol—as we use it—requires considerable preparation, so does heroin but not so its source—opium. Synthesizing or manufacturing drugs—usually by pharmaceutical companies—provides us with refined forms of natural drugs, synthetics which substitute for natural drugs and chemical compounds of new drugs all of which add to the range of effects and our responses to them. Then too, we must include a large number of non-drug products or chemicals such as solvents, gasoline, and glues that are abused for their psychoactive effects.

Like most other things in our world, drugs can be used to advantage or disadvantage. Sometimes we cannot predict which will prevail. An analogy once earlier used is that of the "hammer and chisel." In the hands of a Michelangelo they are used to produce sculpture of awesome and everlasting beauty. The same tools in the hands of someone less talented or an emotionally unstable person lead to different and even disastrous results.[1] Having these tools, like drugs, presents opportunities or advantages and hazards or disadvantages.

DRUGS AND MEDICINES

The benefits of drugs as medicines are documented by the reduction of disease, and improved health and longevity of our population. The search for new drugs continues almost unabated and we read with regularity about the discovery of a new drug "cure" or treatment. In time we also learn that this "new" drug (or new use for an old one) has unfavorable side-effects (adverse reactions) in some of the users. Or perhaps there is a critical dosage with a fine line between benefit and harm or even fatal overdose. For example, lithium is an antidepressant prescribed to restore manic-depressive patients to a feeling of normalcy (not a cure for this condition). First used in 1855 for various physical ailments, lithium is currently being highly promoted by some psychiatrists and a famous show business patient as "the drug that fights depression." Along with other antidepressant drugs, the use of lithium is recommended in popular magazines to "bring new life to your life."[2] However, notwithstanding the risk of mis-diagnosing manic-depressive disease—the particular depressive condition for which there is evidence that lithium can be effective—the careful monitoring of dosage is required to prevent life-threatening reactions. There is also the growing problem of adverse reactions due to the simultaneous use of two or more drugs which interact in a counter-productive or dangerous manner.

Why are we so willing to resort to drugs and run their consequent risks? It may not be the fault of our physicians who too readily prescribe, but of us the patients, too unwilling to endure some pain or discomfort. As a people we may be spoiled by our concept of "the good life" or by impatience to get on with the job—work, move, make, produce! Even tension and conflict—often necessary to motivate us to action, solution, invention, and creation—are conditions from which we seek chemical relief. It seems incongruous.

Exaggeration of the extent to which we are a drug-using society is difficult if not impossible. How are 15,000 tons of aspirin per year produced in the United States (other nations produce it too) consumed?[3] How about American expenditures each year of: $2.5 billion for prescribed psychoactive pharmaceuticals; $2.5 billion for coffee, tea, and cocoa; $12 billion for cigars and cigarettes; $25 billion for alcohol; and an estimated $2 billion for illegal drugs?[4]

The amount of "air" time on television and radio, advertisements in magazines, newspapers, and on billboards is symptomatic of our condition. Are we unwillingly induced (seduced?) to use all the self-medications, alcohol, tobacco, and coffee we can consume? Do we really love wives more if they take Geritol for energy? Can I eat like a glutton or be irritated by my work yet get almost instant relief from Alka-Seltzer? Is Nytol the best way to get to sleep at night? Can No-Doz help me study all night and improve my grades? We should know that a three-year study was announced which indicates that the $58 million a year Americans spend on non-prescription drugs to help them sleep at night or relax in the daytime are spent in vain.[5]

Self-medication isn't necessarily bad. Of the thousands of over-the-counter (OTC) drugs available many of us can choose and use those that relieve minor symptoms and discomfort. We needn't run off to a physician for every little and very likely temporary condition. But we should remember—as should our physicians—that most illnesses do not require medication. Sometimes unnecessary as well as improperly chosen medication masks more serious conditions and leads to a delay in necessary early diagnosis and treatment. Over-the-counter or proprietary drugs should not be used with regularity or over a long period of time. Aspirin, of which we use about 18 billion tablets per year, is a handy pain-killer (analgesic). But over-use or mis-use particularly in sensitive individuals can cause gastric hemorrhage (stomach bleeding) or bronchial asthma.[3] For the most part, it is a safe drug. In any case, we must remember that pain tells us something is wrong and needs attention, like fatigue tells us we are tired and need rest. To block out these symptoms is to remove our "early-warning system." If we are self-medicating and wish to refute the old adage "he hath a fool for a patient who hath himself for a physician," we should be aware of the need for a physician under the following conditions:

1. Abdominal pain that is severe or recurs perodically.
2. Pains anywhere, if severe or prolonged more than one day.
3. Headache, if unusually severe or prolonged more than one day.
4. Prolonged cold with fever and cough.
5. Earache.
6. Unexplained loss of weight.
7. Unexplained and unusual symptoms.
8. Malaise (feeling poorly) lasting more than a week or two.[6]

In any case, following the instructions on the labels of OTC drugs or on the label of medication prescribed by our physicians is important. (See the related discussion in Chapter 8.) Our conditioning to readily accept the use of drugs creates a vicious cycle. We are less attentive to instructions and hazards, and we more easily accept other drugs to counteract the first. A common example is the use of "pep" pills to wake us up and "downers" to get us to sleep.

DRUG DEPENDENCE

Drug use is appropriate when the "proper" drug is used in the "proper" dosage, time, and place, and by the person for whom it is the "proper" drug. Ethical drugs prescribed by physicians, OTC or proprietary drugs, home remedies, coffee (caffeine), tobacco (nicotine), and alcohol can be "properly" used. Too often they are misused.

Misuse occurs in different ways. Inappropriate self-medication—the wrong drug, the wrong dosage, prolonged use—is not uncommon. Occasionally, we misuse coffee, tobacco, and alcohol by taking too much too fast and later regret our misjudgment. A physician might misuse or cause the patient to misuse a drug by over-prescribing or failing to instruct and supervise the patient.

Drug abuse refers to self-administration of a drug which leads to psychological dependence, sometimes physical dependence and abnormal behavior either separately or collectively.[7] In plainer terms drug abuse is the continuing or chronic and excessive use of a drug causing impairment of health, or ability to function at work or in society. Unfortunately, the term drug abuse is still fuzzy and has grossly negative connotations.

Everyone uses, many misuse, and some abuse drugs. Well, nearly everyone uses—there are so few abstainers when we consider the range of available psychoactive drugs. Precise numbers are impossible to develop and estimates may easily be exaggerated, particularly accounts of drug abusers though they are not an insignificant number. Besides, it is most difficult to delineate between use and abuse. We must consider drug abuse on an individual basis. What may impair the health or ability to function at work, at study, or in society for one may not impair another. In younger drug users we may substitute impairment of growth and development or perhaps add it to our definition. We also have to watch out for personal biases which are expressed by our dislike of particular persons or drugs. My use of pot is OK. They use alcohol—they're "lushes" (alcoholics).

For too long drugs have been equated with "dope fiends," "sex maniacs," and "addicts." The physiological-medical, social-economic, moral-legal, and political interests testify to the complexity of the drug-people problem. Attempting to help clarify matters the World Health Organization revised its terminology of "addiction" and "habituation" to "drug dependence." The line between an "addiction" and a "habit" is too unclear. It might be that an undesirable "street person" is an "addict" but someone with more social status on the same drug in similar amounts has a "habit" or isn't even known to be a user. The term "hard drugs" is misleading though it is meant to classify those for which physical as well as psychological dependence develops. The heavy users of "soft" drugs such as caffeine, nicotine, amphetamines, and bromides will often present physical signs and symptoms which make them ill upon withdrawal from the drug.

In 1957 the WHO defined drug addiction as: "a state of episodic or chronic intoxication produced by the repeated consumption of a drug (natural or synthetic). Its characteristics include:

1. an overpowering desire or need (compulsion) to continue taking the drug and obtaining it by any means;
2. a tendency to increase the dose;
3. a psychic (psychological) and generally a physical dependence on the effects of the drug;
4. detrimental effects on the individual and society."[8]

To further distinguish, they defined drug habituation as: "(habit) a condition resulting from the repeated consumption of a drug. Its characteristics include:

1. a desire (but not a compulsion) to continue taking the drug for the sense of improved well-being which it engenders;
2. little or no tendency to increase the dose;
3. some degree of psychic dependence on the effect of the drug, but absence of physical dependence and hence of an abstinence syndrome;
4. detrimental effects, if any, primarily on the individual."

Because of the difficulties in separating the two terms, to cover all kinds of drug abuse and hopefully to reduce the stigma of the term addict, the WHO, in 1964, accepted the term *drug dependence*.

"Drug dependence is a state of psychic or physical dependence, or both, on a drug, arising in a person following administration of that drug on a periodic or continuous basis. The characteristics of such a state will vary with the agent involved, and these characteristics must always be made clear by designating the particular type of drug dependence in each particular case; for example, drug dependence of the morphine type, of barbiturate type, of amphetamine type, etc."[8]

Considering the range of drugs available and the range of people who become dependent upon them, addiction and habituation are less desirable terms than drug dependence. A significant number of those who are into drugs use two or more and sometimes become dependent on more than one. Though poly-drug use makes the matter more difficult, we must nevertheless try harder to change our attitudes and our terminology to reflect greater understanding, integrity, and accuracy.

USERS AND ABUSERS

Why and who uses drugs to alter consciousness or modify mood is too complex to determine with certainty. Categorizing people and things can be helpful for ordering knowledge but too often leads to stereotypic thinking. Earlier we pointed out that drug dependence is an individual phenomenon.

Psychological and social pressures have been discussed as causes or motivation to use and abuse drugs. Those who become dependent are said to have some abnormal psychological need and are prone to deviant behavior of one kind or another anyway. The self-conscious obese woman, the high pressure-intense-hard-driving executive, the immature teen-ager, the insecure college student, the religious freak, the curious—all are eligible to be "heads."

Among youth and young adults much is noted about the need to appear grownup, mature, sophisticated, masculine or feminine, strong, "alive," willful, and courageous. Advertising for cigarettes, beer, liquor, automobiles and almost everything else exploits this need in our population. To prove independence, to rebel, to attempt the forbidden, to accept a challenge are other reasons for risk-taking behavior. In other words the needs for a sense of belonging and a self-image of self-esteem motivate us to behavior we believe will satisfy. Some behaviors do and some apparently don't. Some risks are riskier than others, too.

Curiosity and pleasure are also reasons for risk-taking or drug-taking behavior. Undeniably, some types of risks reward us with thrills that are pleasurable. Some types of drug-taking can be pleasurable—beer or champagne, a smoke, a toke (a puff on a joint—marijuana cigarettes), and a tranquilizer among them. But after all, the effect would depend upon our expectations, the setting in which we participate, the amount and strength of the drug, and our physical condition.

To satisfy our needs some of us are "hooked" or dependent on proprietary items like tonics, relaxants, cough syrups, stay-awakes, cold medicines (antihistamines), and pain-killers. Others have greater needs or have found more potent and thus more toxic and dangerous substances.

Briefly users fall into three groups—though other categories have been proposed. The "situational" user has an immediate or practical purpose: Weight-control pills, or energy pills to complete tasks, to stay awake for studying or traveling; bromides to settle stomachs and reduce gas; and cold remedies to treat symptoms. Without psychological dependence and excessive use, there is usually no problem. Even "curiosity" may be satisfied by this group.

The "spree" users—for thrills or "experience" or sometimes to flaunt convention—are usually a younger group. Some degree of psychological dependence may be demonstrated. This, in part, appears in the kinds of social settings in which "spree" users function. The heavy TGIF drinking party and the week-end pot party are some examples. Because of the mixed pattern of use and "light" psychological dependence, little or no physical dependence develops.

The "hard core" abuser is heavily drug dependent—commonly the "addict." Associated with a strong psychological dependence, if the drug of choice is alcohol, heroin, barbiturates, or related drugs, physical dependence is included. This drug dependent type cannot function without drugs and is usually suffering from some emotional or psychiatric disorder. Unfortunately, those who have a "problem" and try to solve it through drink and drugs now have two problems.

Before we review some of the hazards of drug abuse, alternatives, and treatments, let us briefly survey the major substances used to alter consciousness or modify mood and through which people create and express their problems.

SOME SIGNIFICANT DEPRESSANTS

Alcohol

> "Alcohol may create problems, but also solves and alleviates them. To drink, to enjoy, to live with liquor is for most an important experience. Why some would prefer to achieve drunkenness is not beyond the writer, but beyond the pleasure of liquor."[9]

Probably the oldest and most widely used and abused drug in the world is alcohol. During the drug culture hysteria of the 1960's and early 1970's, alcohol was pre-empted in the media by LSD, marijuana, heroin and others, but it nevertheless was still the "drug of choice" in our society. There are an estimated 90-plus million drinkers in the United States—almost 70% of the population over fifteen years of age. They consume enough wine, beer, and distilled spirits to amount to 30 gallons for each American, including the abstainers.

Alcohol, particularly ethyl alcohol, is an anesthetic—a general depressant of the central nervous system. It appears to stimulate and increase body temperature in low doses (due to dilation of the blood capillaries). A sometimes pleasant, warm, relaxed feeling is followed by disruption and disorganization of coordination, vision, thought, memory, speech, and mood as amounts ingested increase. The feeling of excitement or elation or euphoria accompanied by increased activity, talkativeness, and sometimes aggressive or hostile behavior is due to the sedative or anesthetic effect on the brain, masking of fatigue, and subsequent reduction of inhibition. Sometimes people use alcohol as an excuse to behave in ways they would not if they were sober.

Ethyl alcohol is oxidized (broken down chemically) in the body in a series of complex processes by the liver. As an average, depending upon the size and weight of the individual, the liver metabolizes alcohol at the rate of almost 1 ounce per hour—1 ounce of 90 proof (45% alcohol) distilled spirits such as whiskey or a 12-ounce bottle of (4%) beer. If one drinks at this rate and if accompanied by food to slow the absorption rate, one is not likely to become intoxicated. If, however, one wants to "get high" only a sniff of the cork—the expectation—can do the trick.

As a social lubricant alcohol is the common beverage. We are often coerced by hospitable hosts and we often coerce our guests to imbibe—much to the sorrow and discomfort of abstainers and alcoholics who wish not to and cannot drink. When blood-alcohol levels rise to a concentration of .03%, driving skills can be impaired. When .05% is reached (at about the two mixed drink or cocktail level), intoxication—drunkenness—inebriety is usually evident. The legal limit for operating a motor vehicle in almost all states is .10%. About four drinks on an empty stomach taken in an hour or less and the legal limit is reached—possibly surpassed—particularly in a smaller person of low or moderate weight.

Though social acceptance of drinking makes for a more tolerant attitude towards drinkers with "a buzz on" or those even more intoxicated, a real immediate hazard is the drinking driver. Of 800,000 accidents, about half are associated with a driver who has been drinking. Of over 50,000 street and highway fatalities, about half are associated with, if not caused by, someone "under the influence."

Excessive consumption of alcohol or "problem drinking" involves a significant number of those who continually desire to be in the intoxicated state. They may have a personal or psychological problem; they drink even though their health warrants otherwise; they try to prove how "manly" they are by consuming more liquor than their drinking associates. The problem drinker causes many personal, family, occupational, safety, and health problems.[10] Gastrointestinal (stomach) disorders, malnutrition (particularly vitamin B_1 deficiency), neurological (reflex), kidney, and liver (cirrhosis) disorders are some of the "side" effects or adverse reactions to heavy drinking.

Found somewhere between estimates of 5 and 10 million problem drinkers are the alcoholics. Alcoholism is an extreme form of drug dependence—or in old terminology "addiction." Alcoholism includes psychological and physiological dependence. Withdrawal of the "drug" leads to the abstinence syndrome or withdrawal sickness—delirium tremens (DT's) which includes frighteningly intense confusion, tremors, cramps, fever, hallucinations, and convulsions. Depending upon the condition of the alcoholic, the administration of appropriate medical care, and the degree of physical dependence, there is the possibility of death probably due to heart failure. There are more withdrawal fatalities from alcohol than from heroin or even barbiturates.

The cause of alcoholism is still debated: formerly—and sometimes still—believed to be a consequence of morally degenerate or weak-willed individuals who succumb to the pleasures and temptation of "demon rum;" currently, believed to be a complex physical and emotional illness; currently, believed by some to be a genetic disorder—an inherited weakness or predisposition to alcoholism; and finally, believed by some to be simply caused by alcohol itself—period!

When compared to other drugs people abuse and which have been placed under legal controls, there is little question that alcohol would have been at least as severely restricted from use if it had not had the long history of social acceptance and widespread use. The "alcohol problem" is the biggest drug problem and it is considered to be our biggest drug industry.[11] We must remember, however, that drugs are not problems till people make them so.

Barbiturates

Barbiturates are the second most widely abused depressants. This class of drugs synthesized from barbituric acid includes over two thousand derivatives. Considered to be hypnotic—sleep inducing—in appropriate dosages, they may in lesser dosages act as a sedative or tranquilizer to induce a calming effect or reduction of anxiety while maintaining wakefulness. When abused in continual large doses, barbs or "downers" have the opposite effect resembling alcohol intoxication and euphoria or even a sense of excitation. Thus, they are known as "goofballs."

Medically, barbiturates help to treat insomnia, high blood pressure, anxiety and emotional disorder, and to control epilepsy and convulsions which may be caused by other toxic drugs. As a controlled, supervised, psychoactive medical tool, they are invaluable. A long-acting barbiturate such as phenobarbital is useful as an anticonvulsant and to treat epilepsy. Commercially, it is marketed as Luminal. Short to intermediate acting drugs—in terms of duration of action—have more immediate effects, wear-off faster and do not tend to leave a "barb hangover." Sodium secobarbital (Seconal) or "reds," pentobarbital (Nembutal) or "yellow jackets," and amobarbital (Amytal) or "blue birds" are in the short to intermediate group and are frequently abused—depending on availability. The short acting thiopental (Pentothal) is a useful anesthetic. Related synthetic non-barbiturate depressants include glutethimide (Doriden) and choral hydrate (Beta Chlor).

As in alcohol intoxication, excessive doses can cause slurred speech, incoordination and loss of balance, and quarrelsome disposition. Long term usage leads to development of tolerance requiring increased dosages for desired effects. Overdose produces a typical shock syndrome—unconsciousness, shallow breathing, low blood pressure, low temperature and clammy skin. Immediate medical treatment is necessary—especially to prevent kidney and respiratory failure. Frequently, individuals inadvertently combine two or more depressants such as alcohol and barbiturates and suffer fatal overdoses. Alcohol potentiates—increases—the effects of barbiturates.

Abusers—those who consume more than prescribed sedative doses—might be taking two to five times or even near fatal five to ten times appropriate daily amounts. Such abuse is associated with psychopathology. Continued excessive use frequently results in permanent liver damage. Physical dependence develops and is extremely dangerous. According to the degree of dependence, withdrawal from barbiturates can include psychosis, convulsions and, if untreated, death. Barbiturate withdrawal is considered to be more hazardous than withdrawal from alcohol or heroin.

Tranquilizers

Tranquilizers are synthetic, psychoactive drugs more recently developed. Since the 1950's, these drugs have been useful in the treatment of mental or emotional illnesses. Ironically, the "minor" tranquilizers, from different chemical compounds, may be as hazardous as barbiturates. Physicians at first preferred them to avoid the hazards of barbituric acid derivatives in the treatment of anxiety, to control convulsions, to relax muscles, to reduce heart rate, and control mild behavior disorders. However, meprobamate (Equanil and Miltown), chlordiazepoxide (Librium) and diazepam (Valium) may have an intoxicating effect which leads to abuse. Thus, some of these drugs can be as hazardous, if sufficiently abused, as barbiturates.

The "major" tranquilizers, derived from an antihistamine known as phenothiazine, are useful in the management of psychotic illnesses such as schizophrenia and manic-depressive conditions. They calm and sedate such patients without putting them to sleep and enable them to function better and to be treated by psychotherapy. Chlorpromazine (Thorazine) and prochlorperazine (Compazine) are examples of "major" tranquilizers which are not likely to be abused "on the street" but which must be monitored for adverse drug reactions or side effects. Driving a car while drowsy is an immediate problem with all tranquilizers. Overdoses of meprobamate can be fatal and chlorpromazine requires careful supervision.

Narcotics

Narcotics have traditionally been considered the most dangerous and most problematic class of drugs and for some time been subject to illicit use. Unfortunately, the overreaction to narcotics generated by law enforcement types has unduly magnified the hazards of narcotics at the expense of more widely used problem drugs such as alcohol and barbiturates.

The term narcotic refers to sleep-inducing and pain-killing but the law and thus the public have included other illegally used drugs in this group. Naturally derived, narcotics such as morphine, heroin, codeine, and paregoric come from opium and are also known as opiates. Opium is extracted from the sap of an oriental poppy. Chemically synthesized opiates include meperidine (Demerol) and dolophine (Methadone).

Opiates are strong depressants of the central nervous system and they develop physical dependence in the abuser. They are effective pain-killers, particularly morphine which is widely used in medicine. In addition to the CNS, they also effect the bowels (paregoric) and relieve coughing (codeine). They can induce drowsiness and sleep combatting insomnia, and reduce anxiety, depression, physical activity, hunger, aggression, and sexual activity.

Opium itself is not widely used in the United States. Heroin, a derivative of morphine, an odorless white crystalline powder, is more concentrated and more potent, thus it is the more popular drug of abuse. Physical dependence develops more rapidly with heroin abuse and tolerance (requiring greater doses) more quickly when taken intravenously (by the needle). The euphoric effect, and sometimes "orgasmic" effect, is more difficult to obtain over time and the drug is then taken primarily to avoid withdrawal sickness.

Overdoses of heroin cause respiratory depression and can be fatal. A constant threat to abusers, overdose may occur due to miscalculating the quantity of drug administered or to misrepresented potency of the drug sold on the streets. Contaminants, infection, and malnutrition are some other problems confronting the narcotics abuser which influence their death rates. Pregnant narcotic dependent women can "transmit" dependency to the fetus. If withdrawal symptoms appear at birth and are untreated, the baby may not live.

Most of the natural and synthetic narcotics serve medical purposes. The particular exception is heroin. The laws have traditionally included cocaine as a narcotic subject to penalties of illegal use. However, cocaine is a stimulant and is sometimes taken by the problem people who misuse and abuse drugs for their stimulating effects.

SOME SIGNIFICANT STIMULANTS

The most widely used and abused stimulant drugs have become a part of the world's diet and social customs—namely, caffeine and nicotine. Medically useful drugs such as amphetamines and cocaine, when abused, are included in the "bad drug" category subject to controls by law enforcement and social sanctions.

Coffee and tea are regarded as food-beverages and are used extensively almost everywhere in the world. Depending upon the amount of coffee, the blend, the method of brewing, and the length of time coffee is in the water, the caffeine in a cup of coffee will range from about 100 to 200 milligrams. Tea probably averages about half as much as does instant coffee. Decaffeinated coffee offers only about 5 to 10 mg. per cup. Cola drinks also contain noticeable amounts of caffeine averaging about 30 mg. per 8 oz.[12] Chocolate may contain as much as 50 mg. of caffeine but a cup of cocoa or chocolate also averages .25 mg. of theobromine, another stimulant.

Caffeine is not a harmful drug to most of us and is enjoyed as a CNS stimulant. Several over-the-counter stay awake pills contain caffeine and are often used by students who intend to cram for examinations over-night. In addition to stimulating the cortex of the brain, it stimulates the cardiac muscles and acts as a diuretic increasing urination. Though advertised as decreasing fatigue and producing quick energy, caffeine can produce dose-related toxic symptoms such as insomnia, nervousness, irritability, and excitement. It also increases gastric secretions which may activate peptic ulcers. Some individuals consuming ten or more cups of coffee per day (or about 1000 mg. of caffeine) have developed symptoms which resemble an anxiety attack or neurosis. Nervousness and irritability may be accompanied by headache, cardiovascular reactions including palpitations, irregular heart beat, nausea, vomiting, diarrhea, insomnia, and abdominal pain. Heavy users of coffee, cola, and cocoa combined can often relieve these symptoms by avoiding caffeinism or reducing intake to less than toxic levels.

There appears to be no physical dependence similar to alcohol or barbiturate dependence. However, coffee drinkers often complain of "physical discomfort" when the drug is withheld.

The use of coffee is associated with heart disease. For as yet undetermined reasons, simultaneous coffee use and tobacco use are associated. Whether or not some individuals have a physiologic need for caffeine and nicotine, or psychologic need or both we don't know. In combined use there is a greater association with heart disease.

Disregarding the carcinogenic (cancer-producing) chemicals in tobacco smoke and residue, nicotine is the primary stimulant in tobacco whether it is smoked, chewed, or sniffed. After caffeine, nicotine is the most widely used stimulant drug in the world. In the United States alone there are about eighty million smokers. Nicotine is a fatally toxic chemical and the amount in three cigarettes, if efficiently extracted, could kill an adult in moments. Fortunately, smoking, even heavy smoking or chain smoking, does not produce fatal levels of nicotine in the body.

As a stimulant, low doses effect the autonomic nervous system (which stimulates glands and smooth muscles), constricts blood vessels, raises blood pressure, speeds up the heart rate, and dilates the pupils of the eye. Increasing doses affect the central nervous system causing accelerated breathing rates, dulling of appetite, hand tremors, reduction of kidney function, and a sense of alertness.

Chronic or heavy smoking has untoward effects, some of which are not nicotine-related. Chronic bronchitis, pulmonary emphysema, cancer of the lungs, larynx, mouth, and tongue are diseases known to be associated with tobacco use. Nicotine may be more directly involved in such typical side effects as shortness of breath, chest pains, nasal congestion, fatigue, loss of appetite, and damage to heart and blood vessels. In women who smoke during pregnancy, there is a higher incidence of miscarriage, stillborn births, underweight babies, and sickly babies who may not survive. Statistically, smokers—nicotine dependent types—particularly those who smoke two or more packs per day, are subject to a significantly reduced life span.

As in caffeine abuse, smokers do not appear to develop a physical dependence as severe as that of alcohol or barbiturate dependence.

Nevertheless, in addition to the psychological need, there are indications of physical dependence when smokers are withdrawn or attempt to quit smoking.

Amphetamines and related stimulants are controlled drugs and thus are less widely used. However, their misuse and abuse by "problem users" is often of greater concern than of caffeine and nicotine—even though these are associated with a greater incidence of morbidity and mortality. Perhaps abuse of "speed" is more dramatic.

In the 1930's, amphetamines were used as nasal decongestants available over-the-counter. Amphetamine sulphate (Dexedrine) and methamphetamine hydrochloride (Methedrine) were originally used to treat depression. During WW II, they were used to keep pilots awake on long flights. Since then truck drivers have used them—illegally—to stay awake on long round trips. Thus, they've been called "co-pilots" and "L.A. turn-arounds." Students have used them to stay awake to study (though performance in examinations is questionable) and athletes have used them to enhance performance—and the results are questionable, too. Undoubtedly, they are widely misused (abused) by housewives and executives to counteract their sleeping pills.

Amphetamines are a class of stimulants chemically related to the body's natural stimulant, adrenalin. Thus, they are known as "sympathomimetic" drugs since they stimulate the sympathetic nervous system which inhibits intestinal smooth muscles, excites smooth muscle of the skin and mucous membrane smooth muscle, excites the heart and increases blood pressure, increases metabolic conversion of glycogen into sugar in liver and muscle thus releasing energy, stimulates the respiratory rate, induces wakefulness, dilates the pupils, and reduces appetite. These reactions are similar to those of anger and fear. Medical uses include the treatment of mild depression, control of narcolepsy (a condition of uncontrollable attacks of sleep), suppression of appetite to control obesity, to counteract untoward effects of depressant drugs, to enhance the action of analgesic (pain-relieving) drugs, and sometimes to treat enuresis (bed-wetting) and incontinence. The paradoxical effect of amphetamines and methylphenidate (Ritalin)—a non-amphetamine stimulant—is useful in the treatment of hyperkinetic or hyperactive children.

The misuse and abuse of stimulants is due to the user's feeling of increased sensory perception, greater energy, self-confidence, euphoria, and inhibition of appetite. Injection of large doses of amphetamines—associated with "speed freaks"—is said to cause a "rush" or feeling like a sexual orgasm. Combined or sequential use of amphetamines and barbiturates for the "up and down" effects is a practice of some "spree" users. On speed, users are usually restless, talkative and compulsive-repetitive—for four to six hours.

Continued or chronic use leads to the development of tolerance. To attain the euphoric effects greater dosages are needed. In several weeks, appetite suppression is no longer effective. (Physicians should usually not prescribe amphetamines as "diet pills" for more than three months.) Psychologic dependence increases, the dose requirements increase and a tendency to take speed by injection increases. Serum hepatitis, venereal disease, skin infections, and abscesses are often a consequence of shooting speed. In the chronic abuser, the milder symptoms of tremors, lack of appetite, irritability, and insomnia are often following by amphetamine psychosis. A paranoid state with auditory and visual hallucinations has been observed with as little as a 50 mg. dose. Sleep deprivation is a contributing factor to both mental and physical deterioration. Considerable weight loss due to lack of appetite and the utilization of the body's stored energy and unhygienic life style predispose to a variety of health problems.

Amphetamine toxicity or overdose have produced fewer deaths than publicity would indicate but coma, convulsions, and possible heart failure can occur. Physical dependence is not a factor in withdrawal and abstinence from amphetamine. But several months may be required to restore some loss of memory and to eliminate some mental delusions.

Amphetamines, it has been said, are synthetic versions of cocaine. Unlike the amphetamines, however, cocaine has no medical use especially since the introduction of anesthetics like novocaine—a synthetic. "Coke" was used to flavor Coca-Cola around the turn of the century. The coca bush grows in the Andes mountains where its leaves are chewed by Peruvians, Bolivians, and Chileans for its mildly stimulating effect. Cocaine is extracted from the coca leaves as an alkaloid and processed into a white, crystalline powder before being smuggled into the United States where it is also known as "snow," "cholly" and "happy dust" among other names.

The introduction and availability of amphetamines caused a loss of interest in cocaine which is considered an "upper class" drug because of its cost—about $50 a gram when available. Currently, "snow" is enjoying a revival among middle and upper class users in the major cities.

Though legally listed among the narcotics, cocaine is a stimulant with effects similiar to those of amphetamines. A significant difference is that "coke" powder may be sniffed through the nostrils into the bloodstream—often from fancy little spoons worn around the neck. Injection or "mainlining," like amphetamines, is another way of consuming coke. In contrast, the effects of cocaine usually last about fifteen to thirty minutes or at most an hour. While amphetamines have an effect of four to six and sometimes eight hours.

An intense "flash" occurs soon after ingestion and abusers will repeat sniffing or injection until they run out of the drug. No tolerance develops but symptoms of amphetamine psychosis including paranoia and a crawling "skin bug" sensation can be experienced. For heightened effects cocaine and heroin are mixed—known as "speedball." Depression or let down follows and chronic abuse can lead to illnesses associated with malnutrition and sleeplessness. A significant side effect of chronic coke sniffers is destruction of the nasal mucuous membranes causing sensitivity, pain and breathing difficulties.

Overdose is rare but can be fatal. Infections due to injections, and bacteria in the destroyed nasal membranes are not uncommon. Digestive disorders, loss of weight, irritability, insomnia, hyperactivity, and sometimes aggressive behavior are seen in chronic abusers.

As with amphetamines, there seems to be no physical dependence but psychological dependence is attributed to the intense euphoric response. Animal experiments have demonstrated the appeal of cocaine.[4] They will push levers continually to 250 times for caffeine, 400 times for heroin, and 10,000 times for cocaine! When Cole Porter wrote "I get no kick from cocaine . . ." he was really trying to make his point in the song, "I Get A Kick Out of You."

SOME SIGNIFICANT PSYCHEDELICS

All of the drugs we have discussed thus far, as well as many we have omitted, are psychoactive—affecting the mind-brain and psyche-personality. Because psychedelics are "mind-manifesting"—causing changes of perception, awareness, and consciousness—their use and abuse is primarily psychologic rather than physiologic. Pharmacologically they directly or indirectly act on the CNS and other body systems through inhibition or potentiation and could be classified accordingly among stimulants and depressants.

However, because of their unusual mental effects—the primary reason for abuse—the psychedelics are in a separate group. Other terms describe the range of "experience" influenced by "mind-expanding" psychedelics. Psycho-mimetic refers to the characteristic that mimics mental disorder and psychosis. Psychotogenic means to generate or produce a state of psychosis. Hallucinogens produce hallucinations—sensory perceptions not founded in objective reality. Since distortions of reality rather than complete detachment from reality are experienced "pseudohallucinogen" would be a more accurate term.

One or more effects would be experienced with the use of a given psychedelic. But as with most drugs—particularly the psychoactive—effects are extremely variable depending upon dosages, combined or polydrug abuse, settings and expectations of the users, and health and characteristics of the user. Most of the substances in this category can produce similar reactions though of different intensities.

Marihuana has a long history of use in a variety of social settings throughout the world. Currently, it is considered the most widely experimented with and used illegal drug. Only caffeine, nicotine and alcohol are more widely used psychoactive drugs. It is prepared from the flowers, leaves, and stems of the hemp plant, Cannabis sativa. It is smoked as "pot" in cigarettes called "joints" and sometimes eaten in cookies or brewed in "tea". Some other names are "grass," "weed," "Maryjane," and "reefers." The active chemical in cannabis is tetrahydro-cannabinol (THC). The quality or potency depends upon the area in which the plant is grown and its cultivation. Found as a weed or grown in the United States, the quality is weak or poor. Central Asia and Mexico produce high quality marihuana, thus the name "Acapulco Gold." Hashish or "hash" is the resin extract with higher concentrations of THC thus producing quicker and more intense effects.

In small amounts, as when a "joint" is shared by more than one smoker, mild intoxication like that of alcohol may be experienced. Unlike alcohol, aggressive behavior is rare. Early physical signs are sympatho-mimetic—increased pulse rate and rise in blood pressure. Reddening of the eyes, dryness in the mouth, increase in appetite and thirst, and sometimes nausea, vomiting, and diarrhea are experienced. Larger amounts may increase sensory perceptions in listening to music or seeing colors. Time appears to slow, space perceptions distort, and confusion and disconnected ideas are experienced. Some loss of memory and poor judgment are often encountered. As with any form of intoxication it would be extremely hazardous to drive while under the influence. Heavy use—smoking three or more joints—can cause "hallucinations", panic or psychotic reactions particularly in inexperienced or emotionally unstable types.

Marihuana develops no physical addiction particularly among light users of American quality cannabis. Evidence claiming that marihauna use causes chromosomal damage has not been substantiated. It is not an aphrodisiac—enhancing sexual performance—unless the user "believes" it to be. There is some question that it may reduce sexual drive. A continuing hazard of smoking pot is the development of lung disease as with smoking tobacco. Chronic bronchitis and lung cancer can occur particularly among heavy smokers.

Thousands of years ago the Chinese used marihuana for medicinal purposes. Renewed interest in possible medical uses of cannabis include the treatment of menstrual cramps, migraine headaches, and asthmatic conditions. Marihuana does not inevitably lead to the abuse of heroin. Possibly it may help to treat the heroin dependent who is undergoing withdrawal. Though de-classified by some laws as a narcotic—which it is not—and promoted as "safe" for legalization, marihuana is an intoxicant and thus hazardous, and it is still illegal for public use.

Depending upon your point of view, LSD is the most notorious, famous, or noteworthy psychedelic but no longer widely abused. Lysergic acid diethylamide tartarate is a man-made derivative of a fungus-ergot which grows as a rust on rye. It is one of the most powerful drugs available in terms of its dose related effects. Twenty to 50 micrograms—not milligrams—can have considerable effect in most individuals and it is often used in 100 to 250 mcg doses. It is taken orally in drink or on food such as a sugar cube.

Physical response once again includes sympathomimetic stimulation: increased heart rate, blood pressure, and blood sugar; irregular breathing; tremor; nausea; and dry mouth. Psychologically, sense perceptions are distorted, including one's own body image, "hallucinations" are experienced, and synesthesia—hearing colors, and seeing sound and feeling lights are reported.

Characteristically, there is a great unpredictability of effects in this psychedelic. Severe swings in mood and emotions, panic, withdrawal, and unpleasant body perceptions, and paranoia have been part of "bad trips" or "bummers." Good trips usually require a pleasant setting and a "co-pilot" or "conductor" to assist the acidhead to maintain contact with reality.

Unpredictability, "bummers" or "freak-out" experiences, and "flashbacks"—recurrent trips long after the initial dosage—are among the hazards and the reasons for loss of interest in LSD though some may still be using this drug to attain a mystical or religious "mind-expanding" experience. Though little publicized, LSD is used medically under carefully controlled conditions to treat terminally ill cancer patients, some alcoholics and some mental patients.

Brain damage, chromosomal defect, and birth defects have been reported for LSD users but these have not been clearly established effects. Nevertheless, this too may have influenced its loss of popularity. As with many illegal drugs, impurities, inert substitutes, contaminants, and unhygienic handling of materials create untoward effects. Inaccurate and misrepresented dosages add to the drug abuser's problems.

No physical dependence is identified with psychedelics. Psychological dependence appears to be significant. When a drug of choice is not available, substitutes will be sought. Among the other psychedelics are mescaline, peyote, psilocybin, and nutmeg. Of course, if you "believe," extract of banana peel will "turn you on" since so much depends on your "head".

Discussion of inhalants as a drug in the category of psychedelics is probably inappropriate. However, since we intend to cover significant examples of chemicals abused by people with problems we would be remiss to neglect inhalants available outside of medical settings. Volatile solvents include gasoline, paint thinners, nail polish, and glue which are sniffed or "huffed" to effect exhilaration and intoxication. Continued "huffing" of these substances can adversely affect—even permanently—neurologic motor activity.[13] Damage to liver, kidney, heart, and skin membranes is often a consequence. Sniffing aerosols for the effect of Freon gas has in several cases been fatal. In commercial settings where solvents, glue, and gases are used, individuals who wish to avoid undesirable intoxication and its adverse effects should use masks and other equipment safety devices.

REHABILITATION

For the drug abuser who requires treatment for adverse drug reaction, or toxic reaction and overdose, immediate medical aid is usually available. Some of the drugs abused on the one hand are used to counter-act and treat abuse of an opposing drug. A stimulant might be administered to treat an overdose of depressant. An anti-depressant or tranquilizer might be used to counter-act an overdose of stimulant. A substitute or controlled amount of drugs might be administered to control the effects of withdrawal sickness. This is no game for the amateur pharmacologist or the "sophisticated" drug user-abuser to play. Adverse reactions, potentiating effects and paradoxical responses are a real possibility and require pharmacologic-medical knowledge. Even those who are committed to the illegal use of chemical substances owe it to themselves and their friends to seek medical treatment in hospitals, usually, for severe adverse drug reaction.

Fortunately, for the user-abuser who desires to rid himself of his dependency, there are treatment and rehabilitation facilities in numerous locations. Synanon, Daytop, Huckleberry House, Odessey, Conquest

House, Community Mental Health Centers and Free Clinics are among those available. After treatment for withdrawal or drying-out in a clinic or hospital the would-be ex-addict can join a drug-free therapeutic community. Here the process of helping the individual reconstruct his personality, learn productive skills, develop new habits and most of all establish a new self-image—a sense of self-esteem—takes several months and even years. Alcoholics Anonymous has been successful for many ex-alcoholics. But the key to the probability of successful rehabilitation—which is so elusive—is the problem person himself.

HAZARDS AND HIGHS

After all is said and done, there is one hazard-disadvantage-danger of drug abuse which, though unmeasurable, seems to lead all the rest. Certainly there are hundreds even thousands of deaths due to overdose (Incidentally, there are estimates of upwards of 30,000 deaths due to adverse drug reactions in hospitals).[14] There are suicides while under the influence of drugs and chemicals. There are serious infections of blood, skin, liver, and other organs due to unsterile needles, contaminated drugs, and instruments used by illicit drug takers. There are bad trips, bummers, freak outs, and some permanent psychotic breakdowns. All of these added together represent a somewhat small percentage of incidents when compared to the total number of drug users and abusers. Thankfully, most of us in the user group and a large number (unknown) in the abuser group escape the adverse drug reactions and commonly publicized "horrors" of the drug scene.

The one more widespread disadvantage befalls the psychologically drug dependent who expect to alleviate their problems—find solutions—or escape through drugs. At greatest risk are the young who need to learn to cope; to resolve conflict; to weigh risks, advantages and disadvantages, pros and cons; to choose from alternatives; and to solve problems by working at them. This is an especially important part of growing and maturing. Avoidance and escape through drugs and chemical substances contributes to arrested development—plain and simple. The drug abuser, at any age, is not learning, growing, expanding—though he or she wants to believe he is—but is "standing still." The sixteen-year-old drug dependent is often emotionally a sixteen year old ten years later at twenty-six years of age. Some drug abusers "mature out" of the drug scene at thirty-five or forty asking themselves, "Why this? Where has it gotten me?" After "drying out," or going "cold turkey," or going "on the wagon," many of them have to learn or re-learn how to face problems, function in the "straight" world, and develop legitimate skills and competencies to support themselves.

The social cost—to society, to community, to family and loved ones—is enormous. The personal cost is impossible to place a value on but is of real consequence. Our problem is to learn how to respect ourselves and solve our problems on a more rational basis. Our drug problem is to learn how to enjoy the gifts of nature, the nectar of the gods, and the creations of man. A bottle of wine shared with family at dinner or at a religious feast, an occasional cigar or cigarette, a few tokes on a roach, a cocktail at the end of a working day, a tranquilizer during a family crisis are among the many pleasures and aids available to us at no great health risk—the law notwithstanding.

When we seek the "highs," the "thrills," the "far-out" experiences, and the challenges there are many alternatives. Try learning to fly a plane, skydiving, hang-flying, scuba-diving, tennis, TM, yoga, backpacking, painting, a musical instrument, and a thousand other possibilities. When the hassle gets tough, recall the alcoholic's prayer:

"God grant me the serenity to accept the things I cannot change,
courage to change the things I can,
and wisdom to know the difference."

PROBLEMS FOR YOUR CONSIDERATION

1. Have you used amphetamines for weight control or other prescribed purposes? Describe the effects and your results. Under what circumstances would you consider the continued use of amphetamines?

2. Which, if any, of the stimulants do you regularly use? Why? Are you satisfied with the practice? Do you plan to continue?

3. Have you had experience in the use of depressants including alcohol? One or more? Which ones? Can you describe the effects? Did you like it? Why or why not?

4. Who would be worse off: amphetamine abusers, barbiturate abusers, or alcohol abusers? In what ways is one more of a "problem" than others? Does this relate to the people who abuse them? How?

5. What are the current laws in your community regarding the use of, possession of, and sale of marihuana, alcohol, heroin, barbiturates, amphetamines?

6. Are there "family remedies" used for "generations" in your family? What "home remedies" are available to you? Are any dangerous drugs included in your medicine cabinet? If so, what are they?

REFERENCES

1. Kaplan, Robert: *Drug Abuse: Perspectives on Drugs.* Dubuque, Iowa, William C. Brown Publisher, 1971.
2. Wykert, John: Warning: Lithium Pushers Are Dangerous to Your Health, *New York,* 8:52 (December, 1975).
3. Weiss, Harvey J.: Aspirin—A Dangerous Drug? *JAMA,* 229:1221 (August, 1974).
4. Fort, Joel and Cory, Christopher T.: *American Drugstore: A (Alcohol) to V (Valium).* Social Issues Series, Number 2, Boston: Educational Associates, 1975.
5. Associated Press Release: Drug Safety Questioned By Scientists, *Columbus Dispatch,* Friday, December 5, 1975, p. B-5.
6. Food and Drug Administration: *The Use and Misuse of Drugs,* Publication No. 46 Washington D.C.: U. S. Government Printing Office, 1968, p. 6.
7. Adapted from AMA Committee on Alcoholism and Addiction: Dependence on Barbiturates and Other Sedative Drugs, *JAMA* 193:673, (August, 1965).
8. Eddy, Nathan B., *et al.:* "Drug Dependence: Its Significance and Characteristics," *Bulletin of the World Health Organization,* 32:721 (1965).
9. Chafetz, Morris E.: *Liquor: The Servant of Man,* Boston, Little, Brown and Co., 1965.
10. Carroll, Charles R.: *Alcohol: Use, Nonuse, and Abuse,* 2nd Ed., Dubuque, Iowa, Wm. C. Brown Company Publishers, 1975.
11. Fort, Joel: *Alcohol: Our Biggest Drug Problem.* New York, McGraw-Hill Book Company, 1973.
12. Nagy, Margarita: Caffeine Content of Beverages and Chocolate, *JAMA,* 229:337, (July, 1974).
13. Prockop, Leon D. *et al.:* Huffer's Neuropathy, *JAMA,* 229:1083, (August, 1974).
14. Karch, Fred E., and Lasagna, Louis: Adverse Drug Reactions: A Critical Review, *JAMA,* 234:1236, (December, 1975).

5

Food Choices— Wise or Otherwise

What did you eat for breakfast this morning? Cereal? Bacon and eggs? Toast and coffee? Two donuts? A peanut butter sandwich? A Coke? Or nothing at all? The chances are good that your breakfast, like that of many millions of Americans, followed one or more of these patterns. *Why* you selected *what* you did is an interesting matter. It was quick and easy to prepare. It was inexpensive or moderate in cost. You were hungry. Or perhaps most likely, you just *enjoy* it. Indeed, food *should* be enjoyed, and eating *should* be a pleasurable experience, whether it's a simple sandwich or a fancy banquet. Contrary to popular thought, however, food can be enjoyed, eating can be pleasurable, and at the same time, we can *also* be well nourished. It's not as difficult as it may seem.

It has been well established that humans need certain basic nutrients in order to be well nourished. These classes, or kinds, of nutrients are carbohydrates, fats, proteins, vitamins, minerals, and water. Knowing that these are needed, it would seem to be a simple matter to select foods that contain them. However, since they are contained in different amounts in all of our foods, careful food selection would become an unreasonable chore and require mathematical wizardry. There is a simpler way, using the "four food groups" as a guide, that will provide us with the needed nutrients and will also allow us to eat the things we enjoy. Remember . . . eating *should* be pleasurable.

Before going further, however, it may be revealing to consider what food means in American life. We celebrate with food: birthday parties, wedding receptions, Thanksgiving and Christmas dinners, . . . these and many other occasions help us celebrate memorable events in our lives. We offer hospitality with food: coffee or other drink and snacks when friends drop in, a good dinner for guests at our home or a restaurant. We socialize with food: neighborhood "coffee-klatches" and picnics, cocktail parties, bridge or poker parties, pizza parties. We punish with food: "No dessert until you clean your plate," or send a child from the table when he misbehaves. Food may mean status, too. Steak has more "status" than hamburgers or meatloaf; lobster is considered fancier than tuna fish. To some, food means security, whether it's a baby whose cries bring a bottle or an adult who eats (or overeats) to satisfy emotional needs. These are but a few examples that show food is much more than just nourishment, much more than just a means of helping to maintain good health. Food is, indeed, an intricate part of our way of life, and it can help us, in physical, emotional, and social ways, to maintain the type of life we want. It should be noted, too, that because food is so intricately a part of our lives, food habits are extremely difficult to modify, and eating sensibly becomes a major challenge for many people.

But what does "eating sensibly" mean? And why be concerned about it? "Eating sensibly" involves securing approximately the daily nutrient and calorie amounts that are recommended for one's age and sex. The reasons for these recommendations are plain. Proper nutrition is one of the essentials for good health. We are familiar with pictures of poorly nourished and starving people in some of the less prosperous areas of our own and other countries. That type of malnutrition is readily recognized, but a "hidden" malnutrition affects many people who have access to an adequate food supply and can afford to obtain it. Physical stamina, mental alertness, and one's emotional state may all suffer as a result, although one's physical appearance may not appear changed to any substantial extent.

NUTRITION GUIDELINES AND NUTRIENTS

Except for the oxygen that we breathe from the air and the water we drink, the body's needs must be met by the consumption of foods. Foods have three general purposes. They furnish body fuel which, when oxidized in the body, provides energy for our many activities; foods provide materials for the building or maintenance of body tissues; and foods supply substances that regulate body processes. Many foods have more than one of these functions, and any chemical substance found in foods that fulfills one or more of the functions is known as a *nutrient*. As mentioned earlier, there are six kinds of nutrients: carbohydrates, fats, proteins, vitamins, minerals, and water.

Carbohydrates, fats, and proteins are the only substances that the body can burn or use as fuel to provide energy for work and heat. These are the most abundant nutrients in our foods, and are usually found together in foods, with one of them more richly supplied than the other two. The carbohydrates are the sugars and starches. They usually provide the main source of body fuel, and account for about 45% of the calories consumed. Both sugars and starches are important in the diet, although it might be noted that in many foods where sugar is the main ingredient, there is often little else of nutritional value. Starches, on the other hand, are found in bread, breakfast cereals, potatoes, and other foods, all of which contain a variety of other nutrients. The fallacy of completely eliminating bread and other cereal products when one is trying to lose weight can be seen here; these are foods rich in nutrients, and provide needed energy.

Fats are another main source of energy in the diet. In addition, they provide flavor and have what is termed "satiety value." This means that meals that contain a considerable amount of fat digest more slowly, and therefore prevent the feeling of hunger that occurs when the stomach is empty. Some fat in the diet, then, can help the dieter to not feel hungry, but fat rich foods are high in calories, so a balance needs to be achieved.

In recent years we have heard a great deal about fats and their relation to heart disease. There are different types of fats. *Saturated* fats are a part of meat, dairy, and solid vegetable oil products (margarines and shortening). *Unsaturated* fats and *polyunsaturated* fats are found in vegetable and fish oils. The saturated fats are solid at room temperature, and these are the ones that seem to raise the level of cholesterol in the blood. As mentioned in Chapter 6, cholesterol is a substance that is deposited on the interior walls of the arteries, and over a period of time, may cause a blockage. In the blood vessels in the heart or brain, this could cause damage or death. It would seem that the easy solution to this problem would be to eliminate saturated fats from the diet, thus eliminating cholesterol, but cholesterol is also manufactured by the body itself, and research also indicates that one's genetic make-up, activity level, stress, and other factors also affect cholesterol level. At the present time, scientific opinion seems to support the concept of moderation or a decrease in consumption of saturated fats and a substitution of the liquid (polyunsaturated) fats and oils which lower the cholesterol level.

Proteins are a vital part of the nucleus and protoplasm of every cell. Proteins are made up of great numbers of nitrogen-containing compounds called *amino acids*. Some amino acids are manufactured by the body; others must be supplied by man's diet, as the body does not manufacture them. These needed amino acids, called *essential* amino acids, are supplied to the body by proteins which have animals as their source. Animal proteins, from meat, milk, fish, eggs, and cheese, are called *complete* proteins because they contain enough of all the essential amino acids so that the body can use them. Vegetable proteins from nuts, cereals, beans, and other vegetables and fruits, are termed *incomplete* proteins, because they do not contain all or enough of the amino acids that we need. With a growing increase in vegetarian diets, these incomplete proteins supplied by vegetables are of particular concern. If used in large enough quantities, and in sufficient variety, so deficiencies in one can be supplied by others, vegetable proteins can provide adequate protein. However, since vegetable products generally contain less protein than animal products, it would be advisable to include at least some animal products in most meal plans. Protein provides energy value and is necessary for the building and maintenance of body tissues. Hazards of protein deprivation, involving wasting away of body tissue, do exist, particularly in the developing nations of the world. Furthermore, there seems to be evidence that protein deprivation in young children may cause mental retardation. This problem occurs in some sections of the United States, as well as in other countries.

Would you like to protect yourself from colds? Improve your sex life? Prevent cancer? These are but a few of the claims that have been made for various vitamins. Vitamins *are* good for us; indeed, they're necessary for normal growth and health maintenance. What about those claims? Should we take vitamin pills? We'll try to examine the situation.

One recognized expert defines a vitamin as ". . . an organic compound that is needed in very small quantities in the diet to promote growth and maintain life."[15] These "very small quantities" are designated rather specifically, so we can determine just what our needs are. Although the needs may be small, they are essential, since vitamins promote chemical reactions in the body.

Vitamins are named with letters of the alphabet, and are classified as either fat soluble or water soluble. In brief, this distinguishes between those fat soluble vitamins (A, D, E, and K) that can be stored in the body, mainly in the liver, and others (water soluble) that are excreted in the urine if consumed in excess. Vitamin C (ascorbic acid) and the vitamin B group are all water soluble. This solubility matter has some practical implications. It means, for instance, that large excesses of the fat soluble vitamins can build up in the body, and such excesses have been shown to be toxic, especially for children. It also means that if one's diet usually meets the recommended amounts of these vitamins, occasional lapses will not be significant, as stored supplies can be drawn upon. When considering the water soluble vitamins, however, we need to make these a part of our diet on a regular basis, as excesses are *not* stored. Furthermore, some vitamin loss will occur in cooking, and the liquid remaining in the saucepan will be vitamin-rich, particularly if cooking time is long.

Some of the major functions and sources of the various vitamins are as follows:

Vitamin A. Vitamin A is perhaps best remembered for its role in the prevention of night blindness. It helps to maintain normal growth, and the health of epithelial tissue. Rich sources of Vitamin A are found in liver, egg yolk and the bright yellow and dark green vegetables, such as sweet potatoes, broccoli, carrots, peaches, and others. (Actually, the fruits and vegetables contain *pro*vitamin A, a chemical compound that the body converts to vitamin A.)

Vitamin D. Vitamin D plays a role in the absorption of calcium and phosphorus, so that these minerals can be used in maintaining and building teeth and bones. Liver, eggs, and butter are good sources of this vitamin, as is milk, which is usually fortified with sufficient vitamin D to provide the day's needs in one quart. Some vitamin D is also formed in the body by the action of the ultraviolet rays of the sun on the skin.

Vitamin E. Vitamin E is one to which many special powers are attributed. According to some non-scientists, vitamin E is effective in preventing heart attacks and in improving fertility, but research does not support these or other "all purpose" claims made. The vitamin's function in man seems unclear, with some experts stating it as unknown[8] and others being specific.[1] One thing they seem to agree on is that the average person probably obtains all he needs from his usual diet.

Vitamin K. Vitamin K is essential in the body processes involved in blood clotting. No specific recommended amount of it has been determined, and it is believed that few people suffer deficiencies. Good food sources include the green leafy vegetables, such as lettuce, spinach, cauliflower, egg yolk, liver, and other foods.

Vitamin C. Vitamin C (ascorbic acid) is one of the water soluble vitamins, so care in food preparation is necessary to prevent some loss. Its role in the body is varied, since it helps maintain the health of connective tissue, promotes the healing of wounds, and protects the body against infections. In recent years this latter fact has been accorded much attention, and claims have been made for vitamin C, taken in large amounts, as a cold preventive. The scientific evidence to support these claims is not adequate at this time. There are many excellent sources of vitamin C, including citrus fruits, tomatoes, strawberries, cantaloupes, peppers, broccoli, and green, leafy vegetables. Vitamin C loss from food is minimized by short cooking times, use of as little water as possible in the cooking process, refrigeration of the foods, tightly covered kettles in the cooking process and covered containers when storing juices or cooked foods.

B Complex Vitamins. The B complex vitamins include B_1 (thiamine), B_2 (riboflavin), niacin (nicotinic acid), B_6, pantothenic acid, biotin, choline, folic acid, and B_{12}. Although each has particular qualities and functions, the details are not of major importance for our purpose. This does not minimize their importance. They are significant in normal growth and reproduction, appetite, the normal functioning of the digestive process, nervous stability, and in red blood cell formation. If one's diet is adequate in thiamine, riboflavin, and niacin, it is probably adequate in the others, as the B vitamins are found together in foods. Main food sources are meats, milk, eggs, legumes, green vegetables, breads, and cereals. As noted earlier, the B vitamins are water soluble, so long cooking in lots of water causes nutrient losses.

The purpose of this consideration of the subject of vitamins is to point out the importance of all of them in promoting good nutrition and health. Extreme vitamin deficiencies do exist, primarily in the very poor of the underdeveloped countries, and we still hear of diseases caused by these deficiencies: rickets (vitamin D), scurvy (vitamin C), beriberi (vitamin B_1), pellagra (niacin), and other conditions. In the United States, food consumption surveys rather consistently reveal that many diets contain less than the recommended amounts of vitamins A and C. Although most of these deficiencies are not at such low levels as to cause disease, it appears certain that meeting recommended vitamin levels contributes to one's well being.

There is an old saying that suggests that "if a little is good, a lot is better," and some persons seem to follow this recommendation by supplementing their diets with vitamin pills. Unless medically prescribed, there is no need to do this. A reasonably well-balanced diet in adequate quantities will supply the vitamins we need. Vitamins in excess of need will be eliminated from the body if water soluble or stored if fat soluble. Vitamins A and D have been shown to be toxic if consumed in large amounts, as they are fat soluble and are stored. To guard against this problem, vitamin A in doses above 10,000 International Units (IU's) and vitamin D above 400 IU's are now available only by prescription.

One of the main reasons why we are encouraged to include milk or milk products in our diets is because milk is such an excellent source of calcium. One of the minerals for which specific RDA's have been established, calcium is often found to be deficient in American diets. In children and young people who are still growing, this may result in stunted growth, bone malformation, and poor quality of teeth or bones if the deficiency is severe. If not too severe, the bones may be brittle or soft. Adults don't need as much calcium as children (except during pregnancy or when nursing an infant), but it is still needed, as lack of calcium is one factor in osteoporosis, a disease characterized by bone fragility.

A second mineral of particular importance in the diet is iron, and deficiencies may cause the condition known as dietary anemia if the lack persists for a long time or the needs are great, as in pregnancy or periods of growth. Iron is concentrated in the blood, and has the ability to take on oxygen and later pass it on to the body cells for use in their processes. National nutrition surveys show that women frequently lack the recommended allowances of iron, due to menstrual bleeding. A wide variety of foods can provide good quantities of iron, but green leafy vegetables, eggs, and liver are especially good sources.

Other minerals such as phosphorus, iodine, magnesium, and zinc are also important in body functioning and recommended allowances have been set for them. A well-balanced diet will normally supply the needed amounts.

Water is the last of the nutrients to be considered here, but might well be considered the most important, since a person can live without food for weeks, but without water for only a few days. One of the major purposes of water is to serve as a solvent. It carries various substances in solution, and provides a medium in which chemical reactions between these substances take place. Water is an essential part of all tissues and is also important in regulating body temperature. We often hear admonitions about the need to drink large amounts of water each day. What many people don't realize is that all of our foods contain some water and that water is formed in the body when energy is produced. In addition to these two sources, we do need to take in water or other liquids (milk, coffee, soup, and other fluids) daily. If a glass or cup of these is consumed at least five or six times a day, our water intake is probably adequate.

The Four Food Groups

If eating is to be a pleasure, it's clear that choosing food needs to be something *other* than a search for foods with specific nutrients in them. Fortunately, that "something other" exists and is known as the "four food groups." This plan involves the selection of certain amounts or servings from each of four food groupings—foods grouped together because of their somewhat similar contributions in terms of nutrients. These groups, and the amounts recommended daily, are presented below. It should be noted, however, that children generally need smaller servings, while growing teenagers and active adults may need larger or additional servings. The recommendations are to be viewed as a foundation for a good diet, with additional foods and modifications in serving sizes to meet individual needs.

Milk and Milk Products

3–4 cups (children)
4 or more cups (teen-agers)
2 or more cups (adults)

Meat

2 or more servings of meat,
fish or poultry

Vegetables and Fruit

4 or more servings

Breads and Cereals

4 or more servings

All of these groups provide us with a variety of options, so individual food likes and dislikes can be worked into our planning. Let's look at the groups and some further explanations more specifically.

Milk and Milk Products. These foods are the major source of calcium in our diets and also provide protein and other nutrients. Milk of any kind will fulfill the recommendation, and cheese and ice cream can count as part of the milk. If these are substituted, more than one moderate sized serving is necessary to equal the calcium in a glass or cup of milk.

Meat. Foods in the meat group supply protein, iron, niacin, and other B vitamins. Included in this group are meats, poultry, fish, eggs, cheese, and also dry beans and peas, nuts, and peanut butter. A "serving" is 2 to 3 ounces, and might be compared in size to a medium sized hamburger. Dried beans and peas are alternates or substitutes for meat but probably provide only about one-third as much protein per average serving. Nuts and peanut butter are good supplements, but generally aren't eaten in large enough quantities to make a major dietary contribution.

Vegetables and Fruits. This group supplies a wide variety of vitamins and offers many choices. Within the recommended four servings per day there are two further recommendations: three or four times a week include a dark green leafy or deep yellow vegetable or yellow fruit, for vitamin A, and include a citrus fruit, tomatoes or other good vitamin C source each day.

Breads and Cereals. This group provides a variety of the B vitamins as well as significant amounts of protein and iron. A slice of bread is considered a serving, as is 3/4 to 1 cup of cold cereal or 1/2 to 3/4 cup of cooked cereal (or grits, macaroni, spaghetti, noodles, or rice). Breads and cereals should be whole grain or enriched or restored. That is, the nutrients lost during processing are added, or additional nutrients are added. Most states require this by law.

Nutrition Labeling

Even with effort and good intentions it has sometimes been difficult to determine the nutritional value of many food products, and even more difficult to compare nutritive values and relative costs of different foods. This situation has changed recently, however, due to food labeling regulations issued by the U.S. Food and Drug Administration. Labeling involves providing information about the food's nutritional value on the food packages. Included must be calories per serving, and per serving amounts of protein, carbohydrates and fats, and specified vitamins and minerals in terms of the percentage of the RDA that a serving of the food provides. If a food product is shipped in interstate commerce, this labeling is necessary if nutrition claims are made for the food or if any vitamins, minerals, or protein have been added to the product.

Labeling should make us more aware of the nutrients needed daily, should enable us to detect claims that are difficult to support, and should also help us get our money's worth when we shop.

WEIGHT CONTROL

Weight control is probably one of the most talked-about topics in the United States today. It would be a likely guess that the majority of the women reading this text, and some of the men, too, have been on a diet at least once in their lives.

Our population is so weight-conscious today that diet books are almost always on the best seller lists, magazines carry ads for diet aids of all sorts—pills, reducing equipment and other products, and popular magazines regularly feature diets and exercise programs to help us slim down and shape up.

There was a time when being plump or overweight conveyed the achievement of affluence (the overweight person could afford quantities of good food) or of good health (the plump baby is obviously healthy, or the overweight person clearly doesn't have a "wasting away" disease). But times have changed. Today we know that excess weight is a physical liability and may be a social liability as well.

Overweight and obesity are two terms used in speaking of weight above desirable or recommended levels. The difference between the two is not agreed upon by all, but *overweight* commonly means weight 10 to 20% above the recommended level, while *obesity* refers to weight *more* than 20% above the recommended level. Obesity is a disorder in which there is an abnormal enlargement of the adipose mass. Recent research seems to indicate that in obesity, alterations may occur in adipose cell size, cell number, or both. The type of obesity characterized by increases in cell number is likely to start during the first few years of life, or, later, around the time of puberty. Some cell enlargement may also occur. The massively obese persons are usually found in this group.[10]

A second type of obesity is characterized by enlarged adipose cells, but normal cell numbers. This type of obesity begins in adulthood, and is usually mild to moderate in severity.[10]

There are a number of highly scientific ways to determine excess weight, but for most persons, several other methods of determining it will be satisfactory.

The mirror test. Looking at yourself naked in a mirror is often a more reliable guide for estimating obesity than body weight. If you *look* fat, you probably *are* fat. (This becomes a certainty if you also weigh appreciably more than you did at 25, if a man; at 21, if a woman, and if you looked your best then.)

The pinch test. If appearance does not give a clear answer, the pinch test usually will. It has been estimated that in persons under 50, at least half of the body fat is found directly under the skin. At many locations on the body—such as the back of the upper arm, the side of the lower chest, the back just below the shoulder blade, the back of the calf, or the abdomen—a fold of skin and subcutaneous fat may be lifted free, between the thumb and the forefinger, from the underlying soft tissue and bone. In general, the layer beneath the skin should be between one-fourth and one-half inch; the skinfold is a double thickness and should therefore be one-half to one inch. A fold markedly greater than one inch—for example in the back of the arm—indicates excessive body fatness; one markedly thinner than one-half inch, abnormal thinness.

The ruler test. This test has to do with the slope of the abdomen when an individual is lying on his back. If he or she is not too fat, the surface of the abdomen between the flare of the ribs and the front of the pelvis is normally flat or slightly concave and a ruler placed on the abdomen along the midline of the body should touch both the ribs and the pelvic area. It goes without saying that pregnancy and certain pathological conditions can interfere with this test.

The belt-line test. In men the circumference of the chest at the level of the nipples should exceed that of the abdomen at the level of the navel. If the latter is greater, it usually means that abdominal fat is excessive.[9]

For most persons, excess weight is a result of consuming more calories than are expended. Although genetic factors may play a role, and glandular errors may lead to obesity in some few cases, the major cause of overweight and obesity is much more likely to be too many calories in relation to the amount of activity in one's pattern of living. Frequently, one's eating and activity habits have been practiced for many years.

The discussion earlier in this chapter on what food means to people has significance here. If eating has been associated with pleasant times in one's life, if since early childhood meal times were enjoyable, food was well prepared and in abundance, habits of over eating may have developed. Or perhaps during teen years snacking with friends became an every day routine, or eating during TV viewing added extra calories. Some people eat to relieve boredom or loneliness; others find that eating supplies an emotional satisfaction that their lives fail to provide. So, for whatever reasons, many people develop habits of *over* eating that cause them to gain weight when their calorie expenditure is inadequate.

Even the most inactive person expends many calories in the course of a day. The functioning of body organs, breathing, blood circulation, digestion, and other basic body functions all require energy (calories). In addition, energy is required for all physical activities; the amount of energy needed is dependent upon how vigorous the activity is, how long one is active, and how much one weighs. If the number of calories expended is equal to those consumed, weight will stay the same; if more are consumed than expended, weight will increase. If the balance goes in the other direction, weight will be lost.

In massively obese persons, weight reduction causes a change in cell size, but cell number appears to stay constant. This makes weight control difficult for the person whose obesity has been life-long. Regaining weight is almost inevitable. (This points to the need to avoid overnutrition in the young; a life-long obesity problem is virtually guaranteed.)[10]

A guide to the approximate caloric needs of the average person can be found in Table 1. Persons whose activity levels are less or more than average would need to modify these recommendations accordingly. Another way to determine needs is to multiply one's weight by 15 calories per pound. This is an approximation of the number of calories per pound needed to maintain weight. If one is inactive or very active, the figure could be lowered or raised.

For many persons, however, the question is, "How can I lose weight?" Let's take as an example a college woman who weighs 140 pounds and, according to reliable charts, is about 10 pounds over weight. If we use the formula suggested above, we would take the desired weight figure and multiply by 15:

$$\begin{array}{r} 130 \\ \times\ 15 \\ \hline 1{,}950 \text{ calories per day} \end{array}$$

This means that 1,950 calories are needed to maintain a weight of 130 pounds. However, weight *loss* is desired. In each stored pound of fat there are 3,500 calories. To lose a pound a week (a reasonable rate), it would be necessary to reduce one's caloric intake by 500 calories per day:

$$1{,}950 - 500 \text{ calories per day} = 1{,}450 \text{ calories per day for a weight loss}$$
$$\text{of a pound a week}$$

At this rate of weight loss, the desired weight would be achieved in about ten weeks. (If a weight *gain* is desired, 500 calories per day should be *added* to the allowance for the desired weight). After achieving the goal of 130 pounds, food intake can be increased gradually to maintain the desired weight.

There are, perhaps, some readers who consider a weight loss of 1 pound a week too little, and too slow for their desires. Some advantages that should be noted are that this type of diet can be followed with far *less* change in one's eating habits than might be necessary to achieve a

TABLE 1. Food and Nutrition Board, National Academy of Sciences—National Research Council Recommended Daily Dietary Allowances[1], Revised 1973. Designed for the maintenance of good nutrition of practically all healthy people in the U.S.A. From *Food and Nutrition News*, National Livestock and Meat Board, Dec.-Jan., 1973-74.

	Age (years) From–Up to	Weight (kg)	Weight (lbs)	Height (cm)	Height (in)	Energy (kcal)[2]	Protein (g)	Vitamin A Activity (RE)[3]	Vitamin A Activity (IU)	Vitamin D (IU)	Vitamin E Activity[5] (IU)	Ascorbic Acid (mg)	Folacin[6] (µg)	Niacin[7] (mg)	Riboflavin (mg)	Thiamin (mg)	Vitamin B6 (mg)	Vitamin B12 (µg)	Calcium (mg)	Phosphorus (mg)	Iodine (µg)	Iron (mg)	Magnesium (mg)	Zinc (mg)
INFANTS	0.0-0.5	6	14	60	24	kg × 117	kg × 2.2	420[4]	1400	400	4	35	50	5	0.4	0.3	0.3	0.3	260	240	35	10	60	3
	0.5-1.0	9	20	71	28	kg × 108	kg × 2.0	400	2000	400	5	35	50	5	0.6	0.5	0.4	0.3	540	400	45	15	70	5
CHILDREN	1-3	13	28	86	34	1300	23	400	2000	400	7	40	100	9	0.8	0.7	0.6	1.0	800	800	60	15	150	10
	4-6	20	44	110	44	1800	30	500	2500	400	9	40	200	12	1.1	0.9	0.9	1.5	800	800	80	10	200	10
	7-10	30	66	135	54	2400	36	700	3300	400	10	40	300	16	1.2	1.2	1.2	2.0	800	800	110	10	250	10
MALES	11-14	44	97	158	63	2800	44	1000	5000	400	12	45	400	18	1.5	1.4	1.6	3.0	1200	1200	130	18	350	15
	15-18	61	134	172	69	3000	54	1000	5000	400	15	45	400	20	1.8	1.5	1.8	3.0	1200	1200	150	18	400	15
	19-22	67	147	172	69	3000	52	1000	5000	400	15	45	400	20	1.8	1.5	2.0	3.0	800	800	140	10	350	15
	23-50	70	154	172	69	2700	56	1000	5000	—	15	45	400	18	1.6	1.4	2.0	3.0	800	800	130	10	350	15
	51+	70	154	172	69	2400	56	1000	5000	—	15	45	400	16	1.5	1.2	2.0	3.0	800	800	110	10	350	15
FEMALES	11-14	44	97	155	62	2400	44	800	4000	400	10	45	400	16	1.3	1.2	1.6	3.0	1200	1200	115	18	300	15
	15-18	54	119	162	65	2100	48	800	4000	400	11	45	400	14	1.4	1.1	2.0	3.0	1200	1200	115	18	300	15
	19-22	58	128	162	65	2100	46	800	4000	400	12	45	400	14	1.4	1.1	2.0	3.0	800	800	100	18	300	15
	23-50	58	128	162	65	2000	46	800	4000	—	12	45	400	13	1.2	1.0	2.0	3.0	800	800	100	18	300	15
	51+	58	128	162	65	1800	46	800	4000	—	12	45	400	12	1.1	1.0	2.0	3.0	800	800	80	10	300	15
PREGNANT						+300	+30	1000	5000	400	15	60	800	+2	+0.3	+0.3	2.5	4.0	1200	1200	125	18+[8]	450	20
LACTATING						+500	+20	1200	6000	400	15	60	600	+4	+0.5	+0.3	2.5	4.0	1200	1200	150	18	450	25

FOOTNOTES TO TABLES OF RECOMMENDED DAILY DIETARY ALLOWANCES

[1]The allowances are intended to provide for individual variations among most normal persons as they live in the United States under usual environmental stresses. Diets should be based on a variety of common foods in order to provide other nutrients for which human requirements have been less well defined. See text for more detailed discussion of allowances and of nutrients not tabulated.

[2]Kilojoules (KJ) = 4.2 × kcal

[3]Retinol equivalents

[4]Assumed to be all as retinol in milk during the first six months of life. All subsequent intakes are assumed to be one-half as retinol and one-half as β=carotene when calculated from international units. As retinol equivalents, three-fourths are as retinol and one-fourth as β carotene.

[5]Total vitamin E activity, estimated to be 80 percent as α-tocopherol and 20 percent other tocopherols. See text for variation in allowances.

[6]The folacin allowances refer to dietary sources as determined by *Lactobacillus casei* assay. Pure forms of folacin may be effective in doses less than one-fourth of the RDA.

[7]Although allowances are expressed as niacin, it is recognized that on the average 1 mg of niacin is derived from each 60 mg of dietary tryptophan.

[8]This increased requirement cannot be met by ordinary diets; therefore, the use of supplemental iron is recommended.

84

faster weight loss. In addition, few things need to be eliminated from one's meals; hunger won't be a great problem; meals will contain variety and can still be satisfying. Losing at a faster rate may be difficult to live with, day-to-day, because of the greater changes and greatly decreased food quantities that can be consumed. Dieting is rarely easy, but if done at a moderate rate, it can be *easier*, and need not make the dieter feel deprived, unhappy, or continually hungry.

We often hear people wish that they could lose weight quickly, or we know some one who lost 5 pounds last week. This brings up the consideration of safe dieting. Anyone who is not in good health should diet only under a physician's supervision. For those in good health, it is still considered wise to check with a physician if you wish to lose more than 10 pounds. The speed of weight loss should be moderate, and 1 pound a week is considered safe for most persons. Although we may read about some persons losing vast amounts of weight in a short time, if done safely, they are under careful medical supervision or may even be hospitalized during the time involved. Safe dieting also involves the daily inclusion of all of the recommended servings of the four food groups in one's diet, in order to maintain the RDA level. This is difficult to do if the daily caloric intake is less than 1,000 calories for women or about 1500 calories for men.

Many of the diet books and articles that are advertised widely propose diet plans that are unsafe, unwise, or both. Some plans suggest the elimination of one nutrient group, such as carbohydrates, from the diet. Others propose vast quantities of one particular food and the elimination of most others. Still others suggest extremely low caloric intake. In all of these programs, it would be impossible to maintain adequate nutrition. Furthermore, those people who have weight problems should realize that their basic eating habits must be modified, and that the modification must be something *that they can live with* . . . probably for the rest of their lives. Few, if any, of the highly advertised diets propose such a plan.

The importance of exercise in weight control should be considered, too. The college student who wished to lose 10 pounds *could* do it by increasing the amount of activity in her life. It might take her longer than ten weeks, but it could be done. For example: walking at a rate of 3 miles per hour uses 1.5 calories per pound of body weight: 140 lbs. $\times$ 1.5 = 210 cals. burned in one hour. If our dieter added even a half hour of walking to her daily exercise routine, therefore, it would mean she could cut her calories by *400* per day, rather than 500. Or, if she chooses to maintain her present food consumption patterns, the added walking would result in a 10 pound weight loss in about a year. If swimming or

TABLE 2. Energy equivalents of food calories expressed in minutes of activity. From Konishi.[6]

FOOD	CALORIES	ACTIVITY				
		Walking*	Riding bicycle†	Swimming‡	Running#	Reclining¶
		min.	min.	min.	min.	min.
Apple, large	101	19	12	9	5	78
Bacon, 2 strips	96	18	12	9	5	74
Banana, small	88	17	11	8	4	68
Beans, green, 1 c.	27	5	3	2	1	21
Beer, 1 glass	114	22	14	10	6	88
Bread and butter	78	15	10	7	4	60
Cake, 1/12, 2-layer	356	68	43	32	18	274
Carbonated beverage, 1 glass	106	20	13	9	5	82
Carrot, raw	42	8	5	4	2	32
Cereal, dry ½ c, with milk and sugar	200	38	24	18	10	154
Cheese, cottage, 1 Tbsp.	27	5	3	2	1	21
Cheese, Cheddar, 1 oz.	111	21	14	10	6	85
Chicken, fried, ½ breast	232	45	28	21	12	178
Chicken, "TV" dinner	542	104	66	48	28	417
Cookie, plain, 148/lb.	15	3	2	1	1	12
Cookie, chocolate chip	51	10	6	5	3	39
Doughnut	151	29	18	13	8	116
Egg, fried	110	21	13	10	6	85
Egg, boiled	77	15	9	7	4	59
French dressing, 1 Tbsp.	59	11	7	5	3	45
Halibut steak, ¼ lb.	205	39	25	18	11	158
Ham, 2 slices	167	32	20	15	9	128
Ice cream, 1/6 qt.	193	37	24	17	10	148
Ice cream soda	255	49	31	23	13	196
Ice milk, 1/6 qt.	144	28	18	13	7	111
Gelatin, with cream	117	23	14	10	6	90
Malted milk shake	502	97	61	45	26	386
Mayonnaise, 1 Tbsp.	92	18	11	8	5	71
Milk, 1 glass	166	32	20	15	9	128
Milk, skim, 1 glass	81	16	10	7	4	62
Milk shake	421	81	51	38	22	324
Orange, medium	68	13	8	6	4	52
Orange juice, 1 glass	120	23	15	11	6	92
Pancake with sirup	124	24	15	11	6	95
Peach, medium	46	9	6	4	2	35
Peas, green, ½ c.	56	11	7	5	3	43
Pie, apple, 1/6	377	73	46	34	19	290
Pie, raisin, 1/6	437	84	53	39	23	336
Pizza, cheese, 1/8	180	35	22	16	9	138
Pork chop, loin	314	60	38	28	16	242
Potato chips, 1 serving	108	21	13	10	6	83
Sandwiches						
Club	590	113	72	53	30	454
Hamburger	350	67	43	31	18	269
Roast beef with gravy	430	83	52	38	22	331
Tuna fish salad	278	53	34	25	14	214

TABLE 2.—Continued

FOOD	CALORIES	ACTIVITY				
		Walking*	Riding bicycle†	Swimming‡	Running#	Reclining¶
		min.	*min.*	*min.*	*min.*	*min.*
Sherbet, 1/6 qt.	177	34	22	16	9	136
Shrimp, French fried	180	35	22	16	9	138
Spaghetti, 1 serving	396	76	48	35	20	305
Steak, T-bone	235	45	29	21	12	181
Strawberry shortcake	400	77	49	36	21	308

* Energy cost of walking for 70-kg. individual = 5.2 calories per minute at 3.5 m.p.h.
† Energy cost of riding bicycle = 8.2 calories per minute
‡ Energy cost of swimming = 11.2 calories per minute.
# Energy cost of running = 19.4 calories per minute.
¶ Energy cost of reclining = 1.3 calories per minute.

bicycling were selected, the loss would be more rapid. Table 2 provides further details to show how exercise is helpful in weight control.[6]

HOW HEALTHY ARE THE "HEALTH" FOODS?

In recent years we have seen the development of new food industries which bring to consumers food products that are said to be more healthful than the foods available on the usual supermarket shelves. Some of the momentum for this interest in "health" foods comes from the concern of the public about pollution of the environment and contamination of food supplies; additional support comes from those who fear the chemicals used to preserve or enrich foods or believe that our foods have lost most of their nutritional value by the time they reach the supermarket. Still others look to "health" foods as a means of cure for varied medical problems, or as a part of religious practices.

In reading about these various types of "special" foods, we find different terminology used. "Natural" foods are products marketed without preservatives, emulsifiers, or artificial ingredients. "Organic" foods have these same characteristics, and also are said to be grown without the use of pesticides or chemical fertilizers. Both "natural" and "organic" foods are considered "health" foods, but this category also includes dietetic and vegetarian products, some of which contain artificial chemicals.[7]

Certain foods have been feared or favored for many years, so this interest in "health" foods is not new. Tomatoes many years ago were believed to be poisonous, and the simple (and good) graham cracker had special health-giving qualities, according to its promoter. In more recent years a honey and vinegar mixture was promoted as a cure-all, although the claims received no support from the scientific community.

It would be unfair to imply that "health" foods provide poor or little nutritional value. They are as nutritious as the comparable products on the supermarket shelves. There is no evidence to support the claims that they are *more* nutritious. In terms of safety, our food supply is constantly being watched and tested, so that the effects of chemicals can be determined, but there seems to be no evidence that the American public is being harmed by consuming foods grown by usual methods. Perhaps the most dangerous aspect of belief in the special value of "health" foods is when any one or several foods are relied upon for their curative abilities. There are simply no such foods known (except for the earlier noted vitamin deficiency diseases), and to rely on certain foods to cure arthritis, cancer, heart disease, or other ills is indeed risky.

Another risk in the "health" foods marketplace is the risk to one's pocketbook. Prices for comparable products are invariably higher in the "health" foods store. A recent shopping trip revealed the following price differences:

Food Item	Health Food Store	Supermarket
Pinto beans (1 lb.)	$1.00	$ .37
Prunes (1 lb.)	1.09	.50
Apple juice (1 qt.)	1.05	.45
Orange marmalade (16 oz.)	1.79	.75

Thus, the food shopper is faced with a challenge. In many instances his budget is limited, his knowledge is, at best, incomplete, and his food preferences already well set. Eating enjoyably and also nutritionally isn't as difficult as it may seem. Several guidelines might be suggested:

> Eat a variety of different foods.
> Follow the Four Food Groups Plan.
> Eat moderate quantities.
> Read labels to determine nutritional values.
> Question the value of special "health" foods.
> Enjoy yourself!

PROBLEMS FOR YOUR CONSIDERATION

1. Take your weekly shopping list to a supermarket and record the price for each item, noting the size or weight of each item purchased.

Take the same list to a health food store, and record the same information for as many items as possible. How do costs compare? (Remember to make comparisons on the basis of the same amount/weight of each product.)

2. Keep a record of all foods and beverages consumed for at least four or five days. Be sure to include snacks. How does your food intake compare with the recommended Four Food Groups?

3. Using the RDA Table included in this chapter as your guide, analyze on a daily basis the nutrient values of the meals (and snacks) recorded in problem 2 (above). Determine, also, the caloric intake. Do any foods or food groups need to be added to your diet to increase your ability to meet nutritional needs?

4. Talk to the home economist at your county's Agricultural Extension Service. What guidelines can she suggest for planning, purchasing, and preparing nutritional meals for the low income family? Plan and prepare some menus based on the guidelines.

5. Review the recommendations made by several of the well publicized diet books or programs. How do they differ? How well does each meet the Four Food Groups plan and the RDA's for your sex and age group?

REFERENCES

1. Bogert, L. Jean, Briggs, George M., and Calloway, Doris H.: *Nutrition and Physical Fitness.* 8th ed., Philadelphia, W. B. Saunders Co., 1966, p. 313.
2. Deutsch, Ronald: *The Nuts Among the Berries.* Revised ed. New York, Ballantine Books, Inc., 1967.
3. Frank, Stanley: The Care and Feeding of Today's College Athlete, *Today's Health,* 53: (November, 1975).
4. Frankle, Reva T. and Heussenstamm, F. K.: Food Zealotry and Youth. *American Journal of Public Health,* 64: (January, 1974).
5. Grotta-Kurska, Daniel: Before You Say 'Baloney' . . . Here's What You Should Know About Vegetarianism, *Today's Health,* 52: (October, 1974).
6. Konishi, Frank: Food Energy Equivalents of Various Activities, *Journal of the American Dietetic Association,* 46: (March, 1965).
7. Margolius, Sidney: *Health Foods: Facts and Fakes.* Public Affairs Pamphlet No. 498. New York, Public Affairs Committee, 1973, p. 5.
8. Mayer, Jean: *Health.* New York, D. Van Nostrand Co., 1974, p. 125.
9. ____: *Overweight—Causes, Cost, and Control.* Englewood Cliffs, New Jersey, Prentice-Hall, Inc., 1968, p. 29.
10. Salans, Lester B.: Cellularity of Adipose Tissue, in *Treatment and Management of Obesity* by George A. Bray and John E. Bethune, eds. New York, Harper and Row, 1974, p. 17.

11. Schanche, Don: Diet Books That Poison Your Mind, *Today's Health*, 52: (April, 1974).
12. Schultz, Dodi: The Verdict on Vitamins, *Today's Health*, 52: (January, 1974).
13. Shea, Robert: The Learning of Lunchtime, *Today's Health*, 53: (December, 1975).
14. Star, Jack: The Psychology and Physiology of Eating, *Today's Health*, 51: (February, 1973).
15. Stare, Frederick J. and McWilliams, Margaret: *Living Nutrition*. New York, John Wiley and Sons, Inc., 1973, p. 357.

6

Reducing the Risks of Disease and Injury

For positive health you, the college student, must be aware of how to deal with certain hazards that threaten your well-being. Upper respiratory infections and mononucleosis may cause you to lose valuable study and class time. Certain diseases are risked as you camp and tramp through the United States, Canada, Mexico, and abroad. A venereal disease epidemic is upon your age group. Accidents kill, cripple, and incapacitate some of your classmates unnecessarily. The behavioral patterns you set for yourself today will probably determine your health status at your twenty-fifth reunion. In this chapter, we will discuss the principles for the prevention and/or control of the communicable diseases, heart disease, cancer, and injury with the view of enabling you to pursue activities to reduce the risks of these health hazards.

PREVENTING COMMUNICABLE DISEASES

The prevention and control of communicable diseases depend on a variety of changeable factors creating a need for constant vigilance and research by public health officials, scientists, physicians, and educators. Consider how disease organisms change. In 1957 the type A influenza virus mutated causing a world wide epidemic of "Asian Flu" because everyone was susceptible to the new strain, and since then we have had Hong Kong, London, Port Chalmers, and New Jersey (swine) flu. For the New Jersey variety, a massive immunization program was launched. Consider how a disease organism such as a staphylococcus, once vulnerable to a specific antibiotic, now has become resistant to it. Thus, the development of new "wonder drugs" must be continuous if medicine is to keep its advantage.

Consider the social changes which influence the incidence of disease within a population. World-wide jet travel can spread diseases from one part of the world to another in a matter of hours unless national and international control measures are rigidly enforced. Or consider the fact that in the United States over 20 cases of bubonic plague were identified within a recent three-year period and with more camping and living in rural communes rodent spread could initiate an epidemic.

Consider the many factors that have caused venereal diseases to rise to epidemic proportions since 1957. Complacency is one factor. We thought we had VD controlled back in 1943. In the last twenty years, mass media has exposed young adults to many more sex stimuli than comparable age groups in the past. Young adults have some knowledge about sex and disease but not enough to be well informed about venereal disease control. Ignorance about VD is still appalling. Sexual permissiveness has increased, and birth control methods have changed.

An educated public, technical advances, and alert medical and public health personnel are needed to help solve the problems illustrated by these examples. This section is designed to help you gain a general understanding of the germ theory of disease, to present the basic principles of prevention and control, and to provide you with pertinent facts about some of the diseases with which you may be concerned in the immediate future. Control is better than chance.

The Communicable Disease Process

Communicable diseases are illnesses, the specific causative agents of which may pass or be carried directly or indirectly from an infected person or animal to another person. The agents are microorganisms called germs, microbes, or bacteria which are capable of invading the body tissue and causing infection.

An infectious agent causes illness by destroying body tissue and/or producing poisons. For example, the spirochete that causes syphilis does so by forming *lesions*, or changes in body tissue. The first of these lesions appears as a pimple which may erode to form a chancre at the point of contact, usually on the external reproductive organs, within ten days to ten weeks. Secondary eruptions show up some four to six weeks later and involve the skin and mucous membranes. A long latent period follows. Then lesions of skin, bone, the central nervous system, and/or the cardiovascular system develop. Since the parasitic organism lives with the host, the lesions are the result of changes in normal tissue.

The tetanus bacillus, an organism which can exist in a spore form in soil, is an example of an infectious agent which causes an acute disease by producing a *toxin* (poison). The toxin of tetanus bacilli affects the nervous system of the human being and causes painful muscular contractions, primarily of the jaw and neck and secondarily of the trunk. In severe cases, more complete depression of the nervous system may result in death.

In general, communicable diseases may be considered as having *three stages*. The *incubation period*, the first stage, is the time from exposure until signs and symptoms appear. Knowing the incubation period of a disease is helpful as one can estimate the time range within which a disease may appear after a known exposure. As we have said, syphilis has an incubation period of ten days to ten weeks before the primary lesion appears. Influenza, by contrast, has a short incubation period of twenty-four to seventy-two hours.

The second stage is the *active* or *demonstrable stage*. Cardinal signs and symptoms of inflammation may appear. These are redness, swelling, pain, or sensitivity to touch, fever, and perhaps some loss of function. *Syndromes* (a collection of signs and symptoms) naturally vary with the disease. Some germs attack a specific tissue; others are not so particular, and the manifestation of disease depends on the extent of the infection and the tissue or organs involved. For example, the virus which causes infectious hepatitis attacks the liver. Many hepatitis infections are mild and are not readily recognized; others are acute and characterized by fever, nausea, abdominal discomfort, and jaundice. On the other hand, staphylococcus organisms attack many different tissues and have various manifestations that range from a relatively mild single pustule or pimple to a severe pneumonia or to a rapidly fatal blood poisoning. A communicable disease may be *acute* and develop abruptly, as does influenza; or it may be *chronic*, or long lasting, and develop slowly without a specific incubation period, as does tuberculosis.

The third stage is *convalescence*. The disease by this time has run its course and is no longer communicable. Some after-effects may persist, such as weakness or fatigue. One should avoid complications during this period by taking it easy until full recovery.

A communicable disease may be sporadic, endemic, epidemic, or pandemic. It is sporadic when it occurs at odd intervals and is not persistent, endemic when the number of cases within a population remains relatively constant, epidemic when there is an unusual number of cases, and pandemic when epidemic on a worldwide scale.

There are many types of infectious agents which are known as *pathogenic (pathos,* disease; *geno,* producing) microorganisms or disease germs. *Bacteria* include bacilli, cocci, and spirilla. The rod shaped *bacilli* cause tuberculosis, diphtheria, tetanus, and other diseases. Examples of the spherical *cocci* are the staphylococcus which causes boils, the streptococcus which causes sore throats and scarlet fever, and the gonococcus which causes gonorrhea. The spirochete that causes syphilis is a spiral-shaped bacteria classified as a *spirillum. Viruses* are the smallest of pathogens and cause diseases such as poliomyelitis, influenza, and infectious hepatitis. *Fungi* are multicelled microorganisms that cause ringworm and athlete's foot; *protozoa* cause malaria and amoebic dysentery; *rickettsia* cause Rocky Mountain spotted fever.

The cause, or *etiology,* of each infectious disease is difficult to recall, unless you constantly refresh your memory by using the specific term. You should remember, however, that the science of *microbiology,* which includes the study of the etiologic agent, produces the knowledge most necessary for control.

Transfer of Communicable Disease

A communicable disease may be *transferred directly* from an infected person or carrier to another person, or from an infected animal to man. Infectious mononucleosis is common to the campus probably because of dating-kissing practices. Rabies, a disease most commonly encountered in dogs, is contracted directly through the bite of the infected animal. The venereal diseases are almost always transferred through sexual intercourse.

Indirect transfer means transmission of disease without close relationships to the infected person, carrier or animal. Indirect transfer is possible only if the organism can survive for a period of time outside the body and some *vehicle* is present to carry this organism from one person to another. For example, it is virtually impossible for syphilis to be transferred indirectly since the organism loses its disease inciting power by dying almost immediately after leaving the body.

There are several vehicles that carry germs. Raw milk may carry streptococci, tubercle bacilli, the agents of undulant fever, and other germs. Water carries viruses, typhoid bacilli, and other organisms that may infect the intestinal tract. Food is a common source of germs that cause intestinal diseases. Soil serves as a vehicle for tetanus and hookworm, and air conveys upper respiratory tract disease organisms.

Objects become vehicles when contaminated. Insects such as mosquitoes, lice, and flies serve as vehicles and are referred to as *vectors*. Vectors transfer diseases by inoculation into or through the skin or by deposit of infective materials on the skin or on food.

Natural Defenses

If such pathogenic microorganisms are so common, why is it that more of us are not ill? Fortunately, the probability of disease is dependent not only on the numbers and virulence of the germs, but on the resistance of the individual as well. Unfortunately, the *virulence* (disease inciting power) and the number of the germs to which one is exposed cannot be determined, nor can one know if his resistance is high unless he has been recently immunized or has recovered from a specific disease.

General resistance and protection exist physiologically. The *skin and mucous membranes* serve as a line of defense and usually must be broken before germs can enter. Germs in the nose, throat, and bronchi may be trapped in mucus which is expectorated or swallowed and rendered harmless by stomach acids. The *lymph* and *blood systems* protect us when germs penetrate the deeper tissues. Lymph nodes and some of the blood vessels are lined with *phagocytic* (devouring) cells. The blood carries similar phagocytic cells: certain of the so-called *leukocytes* (white cells) that are capable of moving to a point of infection and engulfing and destroying germs. In certain severe infections the "white count" may jump from a normal 6000 per cubic millimeter to 50,000 or more. The liver and spleen have fixed phagocytic cells which devour germs as the blood passes through these organs.

General resistance may be lowered if one becomes fatigued or chilled. Alcohol in the blood stream may retard phagocytosis. Malnutrition impairs the resistance of body tissue. Many diseases such as colds, influenza, and others may weaken resistance so that *secondary invaders* (opportunists) may get a foothold. For example, the virus stage of a cold lasts but a few days, but other organisms already present in the *host* (person infected) may prolong it for a week or ten days.

In addition to general resistance, there is a type of resistance called *immunity*, which is specific against a particular kind of germ. Certain disease organisms stimulate the body to produce chemical substances called *antibodies* that protect one from these specific diseases. If one has a disease caused by such a germ and recovers, he is likely to have developed sufficient antibodies to give him life-long immunity. This is referred to as a *naturally acquired immunity*.

Designs for Prevention and Control of Communicable Diseases

Prevention and control of disease are dependent on two basically different designs or approaches. One is to build up the resistance of the individual through specific immunizations; the second is to break the lines of transfer.

The fact that some germs stimulate the production of antibodies makes possible *artificially acquired active immunization (vaccination.)** A vaccine contains the actual disease organisms or their toxins. The virulence and number of the germs or the virulence and amount of toxin are modified and controlled so that the vaccine is sufficient to stimulate the production of antibodies by the person, but without risk to him of contracting the disease. Antibodies are disease specific. For example, the antibodies which the body manufactures in response to the modified polio viruses do not protect one from the cold viruses. The *antitoxins* (antibodies that neutralize toxins) produced by the body in response to the diphtheria *toxoid* (a vaccine made of weakened toxin) do not protect one from toxin produced by the tetanus bacillus. You should bear in mind that vaccinations do not necessarily stimulate the production of antibodies sufficiently to produce lifelong immunity. For this reason it is important to receive booster injections at periodic intervals. These intervals vary with each vaccine.

Immunity also can be conferred by injecting into a person immune serums (*antiserums*) which contain antibodies developed in an animal or another person. As the person does not actively produce his own antibodies in this procedure, the immunity that results is referred to as an *artificially acquired passive immunity*. Artificially acquired passive immunizations have definite limitations. Compared with vaccinations they last a relatively short time. Some people become allergic to serum obtained from animals. Unless the serum is administered at the proper time in relation to the time of exposure—which may be hard to determine—it may not be effective. In the case of tetanus, one may be unaware of the injury that provides the portal of entry. Whenever possible, vaccination is preferable. Passive immunity to many diseases is acquired naturally by the fetus from the mother when antibodies in her blood stream pass through the placental membrane. These antibodies disappear from the infant's circulation during the first few months after birth.

---

*Vaccination is used here in the broad sense to include all procedures to induce active immunity artificially.

The following diagram will help you to better understand and remember how the body resists infection.

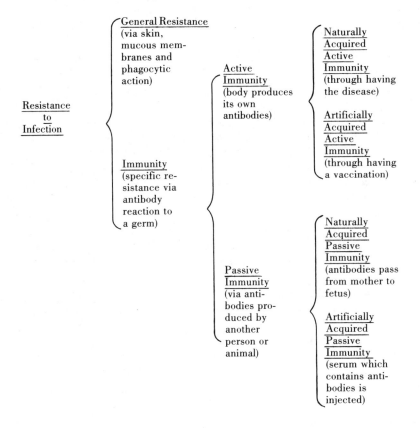

The second method of preventing disease is by *breaking the line of transfer*. Direct transfer of a disease from man to man or from animal to man can be prevented by isolation and quarantine. In *isolation*, the person with the disease is separated from others. Isolation may be voluntary, as when one tries to prevent others from getting his "flu" by staying away from work, or it may be enforced, as when the law requires a typhoid contact to remain isolated until negative tests for the germ are obtained. In *quarantine*, the movement of the known contact who may be coming down with the disease is limited for at least the incubation period of the disease. Because of new vaccinations and antibiotics, this method of control is little used today.

Indirect transfer can be controlled by various methods of *sanitation*. Sanitary measures are carried out at the community level through the pasteurization of milk, purification of water, insect control, food inspection, and other means. For example, the application of sanitary measures such as the improvement of water supplies, proper sewage disposal and treatment, proper food handling regulations in public eating establishments, and pasteurization of milk have eliminated typhoid fever as a public health problem at the community level in the United States. At the personal level, sanitary practices such as blocking the cough or sneeze with a handkerchief, washing the hands before eating and after evacuation of the bowels, and properly cooking, storing and refrigerating food are important steps in disease control. To illustrate, infectious hepatitis is usually transmitted by personal association. The hands become contaminated with fecal matter at the time of evacuation of the bowels. If, for example, a food handler has an unrecognized case, he may transfer the hepatitis virus to food and milk and expose the household to the disease.

In addition to vaccines and antiserums, physicians have drugs that are most helpful in the control and treatment of infections. The *sulfonamides* and the many *antibiotics* have proved valuable in treating many microbial infections. Unfortunately, viruses are, for the most part, resistant to chemotherapy (treatment by chemicals) and antibiotics. Physicians may also use medicine during an infection to support body function or to relieve pain and discomfort. Self-medication for infections is dangerous as it may delay proper diagnosis. When a physician prescribes a drug, he wants to know the physiological condition of the patient, the amount of the drug needed for the nature and degree of the ailment, and the possible side-reactions of the medicine. It was once said that the person who has himself for a doctor has a fool for a patient.

Designs for Action

Designs for action can best be summarized in the same terminology as the approaches we described for preventing and controlling disease: building the resistance of the individual and breaking the lines of transfer via isolation, quarantine, and sanitation.

You can keep your general resistance high by eating a varied and well-balanced diet, exercising daily, and balancing work, play, and adequate rest to avoid over-fatigue. Specific resistance must be obtained by immunization. Artificial active immunization procedures should be begun in early infancy and carried on throughout life. Vaccinations for diphtheria, tetanus, pertussis (whooping cough), measles, rubella (German measles) and poliomyelitis should be completed in infancy. The mumps vaccine is useful for children over twelve months of age and of particular value in children approaching puberty and for teenagers and adults who have not had mumps. Booster injections for diseases vary, but pediatricians and family doctors have recommended schedules which they follow for children of ages one through fifteen. It is interesting to note that as a result of the worldwide decline in smallpox, the Public Health Service's Advisory Committee recommends that the routine vaccination as part of pediatric immunization be discontinued. At the present time, the risk of suffering an adverse reaction from the vaccine is greater than the risk of contracting the disease.

For the adult, revaccination for tetanus and diphtheria is recommended every ten years. In spite of the vaccine, tetanus remains an important health problem in the United States. According to the Public Health Service there were 148 cases of tetanus in 1970. All were people who had never been immunized or whose history of immunization was vague. More than half were in people over fifty years old. More than 60% of the cases were fatal. Routine immunization of adults against polio is not necessary for those residing in the United States as there is little likelihood of exposure.[12] For your best protection and safety you should keep records of all of your immunizations both active and passive.

If you are traveling outside of the United States, selective immunizations are recommended depending on where you are going. Vaccines for smallpox and polio may be necessary. Vaccines for yellow fever, cholera, typhoid, paratyphoid, typhus, and plague are available. Before you travel abroad investigate the public health problems of the country. You should plan to visit and see your physician to get the required immunizations before the trip. Travel agents don't hand out health warnings with their attractive brochures.[11]

Voluntary isolation is important to the health of college students. When you recognize the common signs and symptoms of infection, you should avoid exposing others during the early stages when a disease is most communicable. As you may realize from your study of this chapter, many diseases start with symptoms like the common cold. Your best treatment for the cold is rest during the first twenty-four hours. By staying in your room you provide yourself the best treatment and protect others.

We have already discussed personal sanitary measures that are important in the control of various diseases. These measures need to become habitual. Too often they are underrated.

Communicable disease control by law is a responsibility of local government and is centered in the local Department of Health. As a citizen, you will be interested not only in protecting your own health, but also in protecting the health of your community by fighting for and supporting adequate public health measures for communicable disease control.

We have discussed the germ theory of disease, illustrating the basic principles with common communicable diseases. Designs for action in general have been discussed. At the end of this chapter we present briefly some of the infectious diseases, the specifics of which should be known by college students.

NONCOMMUNICABLE DISEASES: HEART DISEASE AND CANCER

In perhaps no other diseases does a person have more responsibility for prevention than in heart disease and cancer. The development of these diseases and the early detection when cure is possible depend on the attitudes and behavior of the individual. As a college student you may not see these diseases as immediate risks but what you do now may determine your susceptibility later.*

Reducing the Risk of Heart Disease

Heart disease is not a single disease entity. The heart of the fetus may be damaged before birth (congenital) and so is incapable of pumping sufficient blood to the lungs of the baby for oxygenation. Infections may strike the heart at any time, as when a child develops rheumatic heart disease following a streptococcal infection or as when a middle-aged man develops a late disabling manifestation of syphilis involving the aortic valve. Coronary heart disease may result from *atherosclerosis* which cuts the flow of blood to parts of the heart. We have dealt earlier with the control of infections, so in this section we shall discuss only coronary heart disease because the process of atherosclerosis is a disease process which the college student can do something about if he acts now.

In atherosclerosis, for reasons not yet clear, fat proteins including cholesterol, carbohydrates, blood products, and calcium are deposited in the inner walls of the larger and medium size arteries forming plaques. Thus, the size of the blood vessels is reduced and the artery lining (intima) is thickened. This process may occur in the brain (causing strokes), legs, or any organ. When atherosclerosis occurs in the coronary

---

*Much of the material on heart and cancer is based on Cushman, W.P.: *Reducing the Risk of Noncommunicable Diseases*. Dubuque, Iowa, William C. Brown Company Publishers, 1970.

artery and its branches, there may be a sufficiently reduced flow of blood (myocardial infarction) to the heart muscles so that the muscles can no longer function. If a large branch of the artery is occluded by the clotting of blood (thrombosis), death may occur suddenly.

Designs for Action

On the evidence of longitudinal populations studies such as the Framingham Heart Study[7] and clinical studies and observations, risk reduction programs which include the following steps have been recommended: maintain normal weight, exercise regularly, don't smoke cigarettes, heed the danger signals, and have periodic check-ups.

1. *Maintain normal weight.* Obesity or excess fat tissue is thought to be a health hazard in atherosclerosis rather than weight alone. One can be overweight because of heavy bones and/or large amounts of muscle tissue as well as fat tissue. One is considered obese if he is 20% over his desirable weight. So it is important for him to determine what he should weigh (refer to Chapter on nutrition p. 81); this cannot be done by using height and weight tables which are built on averages. The relationship of what foods you eat to atherosclerosis is still questionable. Some scientists feel that a heavy intake of saturated fats is a contributing factor. Certainly for those people who have a family history of heart attacks and have high cholesterol levels, avoiding diets with high amounts of saturated fats would be wise. The chapter on nutrition will point out how you can determine what you should weigh and what you should eat.

2. *Exercise regularly.* The same population studies cited earlier indicate that males who have sedentary living habits are more susceptible to heart attacks than are physically active males. Levels of activity were not associated with the risk of heart attacks in women. Males who participate in high levels of activity may develop collateral circulation which protects them against severe manifestations of coronary heart disease. High levels of activity are also important in weight control.

Exercise programs should be selected by the individual depending on one's present state of fitness, the time and facilities available, and one's likes and dislikes of certain activities. The college student should take advantage of the know-how of his physical education instructors in building a good program to fit his individual needs.

3. *Don't smoke cigarettes.* A cause and effect relationship between smoking and heart disease has not been established, but that smoking is associated with heart disease has been substantiated in study after study. The cigarette smoker has a higher risk of coronary heart attack

than the non-smoker and if he quits smoking, he lowers the risk to the level of those who have never smoked. Smoking may not be related to the development of arterial disease but to the occlusive process associated with *thrombosis* or coronary *spasm.*

Though the reasons are not clear, the risk of heart attacks among heavy smokers is about twice that of non-smokers and scientists feel that on the basis of the evidence collected it pays not to start, or to quit *now!*

4. *Heed the danger signals. Angina pectoris* is the name given the pain which occurs beneath the breast bone giving a person a feeling of tightness. It may be thought to be indigestion. The pain may radiate to the shoulders and down the left arm, usually into the fourth and little fingers. Strong emotion or exertion may bring on an attack. People, particularly middle aged or older people, should report such signs and symptoms to their physicians.

5. *Have periodic medical check-ups.* The thorough medical examination may detect certain risk factors such as high blood pressure and high cholesterol levels and a tendency toward diabetes at a time when much can be done to control them. These risk factors are associated with heart disease and can be controlled through changes in habits and medication.

Hypertension (high blood pressure) seldom produces symptoms that can be recognized by the person who has it and unfortunately it is a major risk factor in atherosclerosis. The doctor, however, can easily detect elevated blood pressure with a sphygmomanometer. He will also check the blood vessels in the eye as these retinal arteries are often the first to show the damage done by hypertension. If necessary, he may take an electrocardiogram (EKG) to see if the heart has been affected.

Cholesterol levels can only be determined by a physician. Studies have indicated that those people who have higher than normal levels experience three or four times as many heart attacks as those with low levels. As mentioned previously the cholesterol level can be reduced, usually by a specific diet.

Diabetes is a high risk factor in atherosclerosis and it is estimated there are over a million and a half undetected cases in this country. The physician during his routine health examination will include tests that can lead to its detection. Depending on the kind and severity, diabetes can be controlled by diet and insulin.

Reducing the Risk of Cancer

Cancer is a general term which covers all malignancies but the steps in risk reduction hold for all types. Cancers are malignant tumors and differ from benign tumors in that they are characterized by a wild growth of functionless cells that can invade adjacent tissue, break off (metastasis), and migrate to other parts of the body to form new colonies of cells. Because metastasis may be initiated early without apparent symptoms, cancer is a most treacherous disease and its early detection depends on the knowledge, attitude, and behavior of the host. Some cancers could be prevented right now if people could apply the art of self-restraint and common sense. You can reduce the risk of cancer substantially by avoiding carcinogens, heeding the early signs, and having a periodic medical examination.

Designs for Action

1. *Avoid carcinogens.* Avoiding carcinogens is no easy task. Carcinogens are the agents that cause cancer. How they cause cancer is not clear, but biostatistics, laboratory experiments, and clinical evidence have shown us that a causal relationship exists between certain agents and certain cancers.

Cancer of the lungs is rising needlessly. It is the leading malignancy, killing "200 persons a day in the United States, as compared to 200 a month in 1930. The present treatments of surgery and radiation are usually palliative at best, seldom curative."[9] Only 5% of lung cancers will produce signs and symptoms that will send the host to his physician. Even with chest x-ray films early diagnosis of cancer is rare. But we can reduce the risk of lung cancer by 80%. *Stop Smoking!!*

British and American studies would seem to establish a relationship between smoking and laryngeal cancer. Primary cancer of the liver is rare, unless the liver has become cirrhotic from the excessive use of alcohol.

Industry can help workers to avoid the hundreds of chemicals they use which can produce cancers of the bladder, lungs, bone, and skin. Protection is not as simple as it would seem since it takes time to learn if new chemicals are carcinogenic; continual exposure must occur over a period of years and the turnover of workers is often too great to allow longitudinal studies.

2. *Heed the danger signals.* The following are early signs and symptoms that may lead one to suspect cancer.

(a) *Change in bowel or bladder habits* should cause one to be suspicious. If one has normal stools and periodic evacuations and then becomes chronically constipated or has loose running bowels for a week or so, he should see a physician. Repeated feelings of incomplete evacuation should also be cause for concern.

(b) *A sore that does not heal* may be caused when cancer cells invade normal tissue. One should visit his doctor when such sores may appear on the lips, tongue, ears, eyelids, or genital organs.

(c) *Unusual bleeding from a body opening* may occur from a breakdown in blood vessels at the site of the cancer. Blood in the feces, sputum, or urine may be a sign of cancer in the colon, lung, or bladder. Blood from the vagina might mean a malignancy of the uterus. There are other causes for bleeding from such openings but when the cause is unknown a medical diagnosis should be sought.

(d) *A lump or thickening in the breast or elsewhere.* Cancer of the breast may be detected by periodic self-examination. The most common involves an enlargement of a gland, and if the lump is caught when small, the cancer can be cured. Since cancer of the breast that has spread may show up in the armpit, lumps there must be checked. Growths on the border of skin and the lip where a smoker holds his pipe may be malignant. Lumps on the tongue or in the groin should be viewed with suspicion, also.

(e) *Persistent hoarseness or cough.* Fortunately, symptoms of the larynx appear early but unfortunately many people ignore them until too late. If caught early, cancer of the larynx can be treated without removing the voice box. Early signs include prolonged hoarseness which comes from growths on the cords. If the cancer is elsewhere, a pain on swallowing, coughing, or a "lump in the throat" feeling may be the signs and symptoms.

(f) *Persistent indigestion* which lasts for a period of more than two weeks no matter how mild or vague the pain or discomfort should be diagnosed. Other signs such as blood in the stool and vomiting often come months later when the cancer has grown and spread to nearby lymph glands or the liver.

(g) *A change in the size of warts or moles.* The vast majority of moles and skin blemishes are benign. They are genetic in origin and appear more frequently as one gets older. Moles in situations where they are constantly irritated should be removed. Others should be checked out if there is bleeding, itching or pain as well as change in size or shape.

3. *Periodic medical examinations.* In people over thirty the family doctor and dentist are keeping the possibility of cancer in mind during patients' regular check-ups. The dentist will look for the signs and symptoms of oral cancer mentioned above, particularly sores and lumps on the lips, tongue, and cheeks. The family physician may use many techniques including a simple *rectal* examination to discover cancer of the rectum, prostate gland, and lower colon. He may use a long handled mirror to look for malignancies of the larynx. A vaginal smear called the Pap test should be an annual procedure for adult women.

Not all cancers can be detected by routine physical examinations. The family physician may recommend other procedures when necessary. The "protco" should be given yearly to all over forty. In this examination the physician inserts a light into the rectum and lower intestines to examine the walls for precancerous growths. Unfortunately, many people refuse such a test as there is some discomfort, or they are afraid the doctor may find something; yet three out of four deaths from cancer of the colon could be avoided by early detection.

New tests are being used such as x-ray mammography to discover breast cancer and new tools are being developed such as a new flexible bronchoscope for detecting cancer of the esophagus and lungs. Virus research is still proceeding at a rapid pace so in the future we may have immunizations to prevent certain cancers. Even with such advances the prevention and early detection of cancer will remain your responsibility.

ACCIDENTS AND INJURY

Whatever you will be doing—driving, bicycling, motorcycling, swimming, skiing, playing touch football, softball, tennis, golfing, or just fooling around the house or apartment—you won't necessarily be thinking about safety. But it is while you're involved in these kinds of activities that accidents and injuries can happen. Accidents are the leading cause of death and disability among college students. We do not wish to overwhelm you with statistics of each and every accident and spoil the fun of living, but rather give you a model of how accidents and injuries occur which may enable you to do something about reducing the risks.

Reducing the Risks of Accidents and Injury

Accidents happen because of an unplanned event that occurs in the inter-relations between a host, agent, and the environment. The *host* is the person involved. The *agent* is the object, such as a car, knife, or poison. The *environment* includes all elements involved in the interaction such as time, place, and physical and social factors. This framework or epidemiological model has provided researchers with a system for describing and analyzing accidents with a view to developing procedures for prevention.* We will discuss the human factors in relation to the agent and environment so you can identify your personal responsibility in accident prevention.

*For a detailed discussion of the epidemiology of accidents read reference 6, Chapter 3.

Designs for Action

1. *Realize your age.* The young adult is susceptible to accidents because of characteristics of his age. He has yet to learn how to control those emotions discussed in Chapter Two. He accepts the challenge of a drag race because he's afraid he'll be called "chicken" if he doesn't. She hits up onto the golf green before the foursome leaves because she's mad at the slow play. Or he dives off the limb of a tree into the pool to show how brave he is. Recognize that your sensory keenness, reaction time, and motor skills are at their peak, but also realize that immaturity and inexperience in many new things you may have a chance to do in college demand a thoughtful approach.

2. *Learn the skills.* Education is important in preventing accidents and injury. Education has been quite successful in reducing the accident rate of new drivers. Laboratories and shops teach specific skills in handling tools and equipment to reduce risks of injury. In certain sports such as skiing it's important to learn how to fall. You need specific instructions in how to use scuba diving equipment. There are many home skills that have to be learned, too. Many people sustain backstrain because they don't know how to open a window or pull weeds; and how about knowing how to use that power mower correctly and effectively?

3. *Recognize that fatigue and emotional states* make you more accident prone. Fatigue reduces alertness, skill, and judgment. A quick nap will often restore your alertness for driving. Change drivers periodically on a long drive. Taking a rest before finishing a friendly game of tennis may prevent sprains, strains, and falls. Know your limits before accepting a challenging swim or before beginning an exercise program.

As mentioned above, the emotions of younger people are usually less subdued than those of adults. That anger, fear, and anxieties affect performance is well known, but the exact relationship of these to specific kinds of accidents has yet to be well researched.

4. *Use drugs wisely.* A variety of drugs taken as medicines may influence safety either directly or by side effects. The relation of alcohol to driving and industrial accidents has been well documented. The effects of marihuana on neuromuscular skills are being studied. The chapter on drugs discusses their use in some detail.

5. *Recognize the inciting agent.* Many accidents may be prevented simply by decreasing the hazardous interaction between host and the agent. For example, confining drugs to the medicine cabinet, putting the tools away to keep them from becoming toys for kids, wearing goggles

when using the drill or putting a mouthpiece between you and the butt of that hockey stick. Though you may not have much to do with it personally, the design of equipment is important for safety. For example, the designs for football and hockey helmets have been improved to reduce head injuries. You may find one bike less expensive than another, but the lower cost may be due to the inferior construction of the wheels or brakes, vital parts for safe operation. The new safety features on cars required of automobile manufacturers in recent years are known to most of you. Do you use these features habitually when driving?

6. *Recognize the hazardous conditions of the environment.* Have you ever come to school on icy streets? Do you take time to defrost all your car windows? Atmospheric variables affect the conditions for driving. Do you modify your driving habits to accommodate for them? In hot, humid weather, do you rest more frequently and quench your thirst when playing tennis or golf?

Your social environment may be a factor in safety. Are your companions risk-taking persons that lead you to unsafe behavior? It's interesting to see young men wearing helmets and mouth pieces in football and hockey today when in the early 1930's it was "masculine" to go bareheaded in football and risk having your front teeth knocked out in hockey. Do you think men who wear such protective equipment are less masculine than those who don't? Do you set a style of courteous driving for others to follow?

7. *Keep physically fit.* Coaches and trainers of college teams realize that conditioning is most important for the prevention of injury. The athlete has to spend hours each week strengthening the muscles to improve stability of the joints and back. One only has to watch the "pros" to realize that conditioning is the only thing that enables them to stand the knocks of the game. Muscular and cardiorespiratory power is necessary to prevent the fatigue mentioned earlier. Yost reports that at North Country School at Lake Placid, New York, 7 fractures and 5 sprains occurred in a total of 5,000 boy and girl skiing hours. After adopting a pre-ski conditioning program there were no fractures or sprains reported within the same period.[13] The person who is reasonably well conditioned will have enough strength, power, and flexibility to prevent injury when being thrown off-balance, slipping on icy streets, stubbing a toe or taking a fall during a sport.

The causes of accidents are to be found in the interaction of host, agent, and variables in the environment, and when you understand the human factors involved in the interrelationships, you are in a position to reduce the risk of personal injury.

SOME COMMON COMMUNICABLE DISEASES*

Common Cold

1. *Identification.* Acute catarrhal infection of upper respiratory tract characterized by inflamed nose and throat. Rise in temperature uncommon. Chilly sensation with runny nose and general indisposition usual. If general indisposition is marked, sometimes the word "grippe" is used. Runny discharge becomes *purulent* (contains pus) later, due to invasion by secondary germs which prolong cold. Spread of the cold to sinuses, lower respiratory tract and middle ear is not uncommon.

2. *Cause and transfer.* Fifty or more viruses cause resistance of mucous membrane to be lowered so secondary bacteria get a foothold. Transfer is direct by coughing, sneezing, kissing; indirect by commonly handled and freshly soiled articles.

3. *Prevention and control.* (a) Keep general resistance high; good diet, avoid fatigue, exposure to chilling and excessive use of alcohol; (b) no known specific effective immunization; (c) protect others, particularly the very young and old, from catching your cold by staying away from them as much as possible. Follow personal sanitary procedures such as covering nose and mouth when coughing or sneezing. Dispose of handkerchief and tissue properly; (d) avoid complications by rest during early stages and avoiding violent nose blowing. Children should be taught to wipe, not blow, the nose. Violent blowing tends to spread infection to sinuses and middle ear; (e) specific treatment: none; rest during early stages may reduce severity. Many persons have one to six colds yearly. The incidence is highest in families with young children.

Influenza

1. *Identification.* Characterized by sudden onset, fever for one to six days, runny nose, chills, aches and pains in back and limbs, sore throat, and dry cough. Usually self-limiting with recovery in two to seven days. Complications such as bronchitis and pneumonia not uncommon among very young and old and persons debilitated with heart and kidney disease. Persons who contract the disease should avoid complications by not over-doing during the convalescent stage.

2. *Cause and transfer.* Several different types and strains of virus, some of which have been identified. New types may occur through

*Much of the information in this section is based on *Control of Communicable Diseases in Man.* 11th Ed., 1970—an official report of the American Public Health Association, Abram S. Benenson, M.D., editor.

mutation. Few people have immunity to new types, so epidemics occur. Transfer is by discharges from nose and mouth and freshly contaminated articles; probably air-borne among crowded populations in an enclosed space such as a school bus.

3. *Prevention and control.* (a) Active immunization the only known method. Vaccines for some strains of virus available, but routine immunization of general population is not recommended with the exception of the 1976 type termed New Jersey (swine) flu; (b) personal sanitary measures in relation to coughing and sneezing in close presence of others should be observed. Avoid common use of drinking glasses, towels, and other personal articles; avoid crowds during epidemics; (c) specific treatment: none. Antibiotics not useful if disease is uncomplicated.

Gonorrhea

1. *Identification.* In males, a thick yellow discharge from the penis and smarting sensation during urination appear three to nine days after exposure. Infection is usually self-limited, but may spread to posterior urethra and cause prostatitis and epididymitis; a chronic carrier state occurs if not treated. In the female there are three stages: (1) a few days after exposure an inflammation of the cervix and urethra which may be so mild as to go unnoticed; (2) a stage of pelvic invasion with symptoms of infection; (3) a stage of residual and often chronic infection. One can become reinfected.

2. *Cause and transfer.* Gonococcus transmitted in adults by sexual intercourse and sodomy.

3. *Prevention and control:* (a) Avoid clandestine sexual promiscuity; (b) use methods of personal prophylaxis before, during, and after exposure; (c) get immediate specific treatment; antibiotics under medical supervision; (d) report contacts to public health authorities; (e) add silver nitrate solution or antibiotic agents to eyes of babies at birth.

Syphilis

1. *Identification.* Primary lesion (a papule or pimple) which may become an ulcerous chancre at point of entry about three weeks after exposure. Infection without chancre is fairly frequent. The primary lesion is followed about five weeks to as long as twelve months later by mild constitutional symptoms and secondary lesions of skin and mucous membranes. The lesions eventually heal regardless of treatment, but may recur during first five years after infection. Late

manifestations occur in cardiovascular and central nervous systems. One can become reinfected.

2. *Cause and transfer.* Spirochete transferred chiefly through sexual intercourse, sodomy, and occasionally kissing during secondary stages. Indirect transfer negligible. Prenatal infection of fetus may occur after fourth month of pregnancy.

3. *Prevention and control.* (a) Congenital syphilis of fetus can be prevented by treatment of the mother; (b) other measures similar to gonorrhea.

Infectious Mononucleosis

1. *Identification.* Fever, enlargement of lymph glands, throat involvement, enlargement of spleen. Fever usually present, but previously mentioned signs may not be.

2. *Cause and transfer.* A virus. Probably person to person, spread by an oral-pharyngeal route. Kissing may facilitate spread among young adults.

3. *Prevention and control:* (a) Keep general resistance high; (b) specific treatment: none. If spleen has been involved, contact sports with a risk of injury to the organ should be avoided during convalescence.

Infectious Hepatitis*

1. *Identification.* Acute infection characterized by fever, nausea, general discomfort and followed by jaundice. Many infections mild and without jaundice.

2. *Cause and transfer.* Virus transferred through intimate person to person contact by fecal-oral route with respiratory spread possible; also transfusion of whole blood from infected person. Epidemics have been related to contaminated food, water, milk, and, in drug use, contaminated needles.

3. *Prevention and control.* (a) Good sanitary and personal health practices such as washing hands in soap and hot water immediately after voiding bowels and always before eating. Keep hands and unclean articles away from mouth. Avoid exposure to spray from mouth and nose. Wash hands thoroughly after handling a sick person or his belongings; (b) specific treatment: *none.*

---

*Infectious hepatitis and serum hepatitis are clinically indistinguishable. Both may be spread by use of syringes or needles contaminated by traces of blood from an infected person.

Tetanus

1. *Identification.* Characterized by painful muscle contractions, first of jaw and neck muscles and then of trunk. Mortality averages about 35%.

2. *Cause and transfer.* Toxin of tetanus bacillus. Spores of germ enter through injury, usually a puncture wound. Injury can be so slight that it might go unnoticed. Spore form of bacillus resides in soil.

3. *Prevention and control:* (a) Active immunization with toxoid beginning in infancy and reinforcing (booster) injections periodically or at time of wound. Vaccination gives protection if injury is unnoticed; (b) passive immunity available if person not protected but has disadvantages of allergic reactions for some people; (c) specific treatment: tetanus antitoxin and penicillin.

PROBLEMS FOR YOUR CONSIDERATION

1. Identify and describe the nature of the communicable diseases common to your age group and set up methods of prevention and control for each.

2. What communicable diseases might you expect to find in traveling through Mexico? India? Africa? What precautions must you take to reduce the risk of contracting them?

3. Circulatory diseases other than those caused by atherosclerosis are common. Identify them and discuss their prevention and control.

4. Such disease problems as diabetes, emphysema, epilepsy and allergies have not been discussed in this chapter. What is the nature of these noncommunicable diseases? How can we reduce the risk of having them?

5. Select two of your favorite recreational activities and analyze (using the epidemiological model) what your responsibilities are in reducing the risk of injury while participating in them.

6. Using the epidemiological approach, investigate two recent campus accidents to learn the cause and contributing factors. Could the accidents or injuries have been prevented? How?

REFERENCES

1. Astor, Gerald: Plague, American Style, *Today's Health*, 50: (August, 1972).
2. Berland, Ted: Coping With Emphysema, *Today's Health*, 50: (November, 1972).
3. Carpenter, Philip L.: *Microbiology*. Philadelphia, W. B. Saunders Co., 1972.
4. Cushman, Wesley P.: *Reducing the Risk of Noncommunicable Diseases*. Dubuque, Iowa, William C. Brown Company, 1970.
5. *Control of Communicable Diseases in Man*. 11th Ed., Abram S. Benenson, M.D. (Editor). New York, American Public Health Association, 1970.
6. Halsey, Maxwell N., Editor: *Accident Prevention*. New York, McGraw-Hill Book Company, 1961.
7. Kannel, William B.: *Habits and Coronary Heart Disease*. The Framingham Study (Public Health Service Pamphlet No. 1515). U.S. Government Printing Office, 1966.
8. Kogan, Benjamin A., M.D.: *Health: Man in a Changing Environment*. 2nd Ed., New York, Harcourt Brace Jovanovich, Inc., 1974, Chapters 8, 9, 10.
9. Neimark, Paul: Progress Report in the Battle Against Cancer, *Today's Health*, 50: 41, (July, 1972).
10. Safran, Claire: Those Summer Allergies, *Today's Health*, 51: (July, 1973).
11. Schanche, Don A. The Health Risks Travel Agents Won't Tell you About, *Today's Health*, 51:54, (March, 1973).
12. Vaccines: An Update, *FDA Consumer*, 24:(December, 1973—January, 1974).
13. Yost, Charles Peter: Total Fitness and Prevention of Accidents, *JOHPER*, 45:32, (March, 1967).

7

Improving Environmental Health

Today, the primary force affecting the life of every other creature on earth is man. And man with his powerful technology can, for the first time in history, destroy the planet's living condition either wantonly or unwontedly. We have reached the point where each human must give increasing attention to improving and conserving the earth's resources and reducing the accumulation of wastes. It is a personal challenge. It is a real challenge and one which mandates some design, if it is to succeed.

Man and all other organisms on this planet live in a "closed system." This *ecosystem* is limited to the planet Earth and its atmosphere, which extends approximately 7½ miles upward. Within this ecosystem are all the essential elements necessary to man: carbon, oxygen, hydrogen, and nitrogen. Also present are all the living and non-living components of the earth. They are all in a state of dynamic balance, and their balance has been maintained through cyclic processes. Consider the cyclic process involving oxygen and carbon dioxide. Green plants are man's main source of oxygen. Man, on the other hand, produces carbon dioxide as a waste product. Plants, while carrying out the processes of photosynthesis, consume CO_2 and produce O_2. One acre of beech forest yields 1,500 pounds of pure oxygen a year, while removing 2,000 pounds of carbon dioxide. One can imagine the enormity of the disaster if this cyclic process is thrown off balance.

For a long period of time man existed within the pattern of things.

He held that the land belongs to all who use it and use is determined by need. His attempts at use were primitive, his numbers few, and, in view of the enormous store of resources which were locked up within the earth, he caused little harm to the ecosystem.

As man's numbers and knowledge increased, his activities began to shape the environment rather than be shaped by it. He exploited the "unlimited" resources of the earth with little regard for the future. It is only recently that man has come to realize that the earth's resources are limited and that their over-exploitation could lead to a momentous natural catastrophe. Certain life supporting cycles have already experienced a shift in balance—a prelude to natural catastrophe if not caught in time.

Aldous Huxley wrote: "Do we plan to live on this planet in symbiotic harmony with our environment? Or preferring to be wantonly stupid, shall we choose to live like murderers and suicidal parasites that kill their host and so destroy themselves." The environmental problem has grown out of the way *we* live. It is a problem of values; it is clearly a problem of priority since the quality of life in the future requires action now.

OVERPOPULATION

Uncontrolled human fertility poses a greater threat to our future well-being and individual security than any other single factor. It is estimated that the world population will nearly double by the turn of the century. This doubling of the world population is occurring simultaneously with a scarcity of energy fuels, an inadequate food supply, and growing social unrest.

Information available for the first half of the 1970's reveals some disturbing trends in the world food economy. During this time period the world demand for food expanded by both a rising affluence and rapid population growth. We are witnessing a disaster predicted by Thomas Robert Malthus in 1798 when he wrote in his paper "An Essay on the Principles of Population" the following:

> "I think I may fairly make two postulata.
> First, that food is necessary to the existence of man.
> Secondly, that the passion between the sexes is necessary, and will remain nearly in its present state.
> These two laws ever since we have had any knowledge of mankind, appear to have fixed laws of our nature; and we have not hitherto seen any alteration in them, since we have no reason to conclude that they will ever cease to be what they now are. . . .
> Assuming then, my postulata as granted I say, that the power

of population is indefinitely greater than the power in the earth
to produce subsistence for man.

Population when unchecked, increases in a geometrical ratio.
Subsistence increases only in an arithmetical ratio. A slight
acquaintance with numbers will show the immensity of the first
power in comparison of the second.

By that law of our nature which makes food necessary to the
life of man, the effects of these two unequal powers must be kept
equal."

Present population statistics are frightening. It took from the
beginning of time to 1830 to produce the first billion people; it took a
century (1830-1930) to produce the next billion. The third billion
appeared in a short thirty years (1930-1960) and the fourth billion is now
with us.

Although the population statistics are awesome, it is more dis-
couraging to consider the fate of individuals and nations caught in the
growing wave of humanity. Unemployment, inadequate housing, poor
health care, malnutrition, increased mental disorders, resource exhaus-
tion, civil disorder, environmental pollution, and a host of other health
problems pose genuine threats to human welfare. Unless the entire
community of nations embarks on a concerted effort to avert chaos, life
in most of the world will become a fight for existence on a benighted
earth long before the last grain of rice is consumed. Individually, the
problem has another personal dimension. In his book *Psychology of
Birth Planning*, Pohlman points out that "if a planet faces over or under
population, it is important only as it affects the lives of other individual
human beings . . . the parent, other siblings . . . other people. All births
are the direct cause of the behavior of individual parents. Any social
forces that influence birth planning . . . can be so only as they are
channeled through the individual."[7]

It is quite clear that any humane program of population control
rests with the individual, his values, attitudes and behavior. The real
hope is in the development in man of an ecological conscience, based on
the concern for the quality of life.

Of course, an alternative to the population problem is to let Nature
solve it her way, through pollution, pestilence, or mass starvation.

AIR POLLUTION

Such dramatic episodes in this century, as in the Meuse Valley
(1930), Donora, Pennsylvania (1948), and London (1952), have demonstrated that community air pollution can result in a considerable loss of
life and serious illness. While the exact nature of the associations

between air pollution and human health have not been fully established, there are some valid conclusions that can be recorded.

It is well documented that the "portable air pollution," that is, the cigarette, if smoked over a period of years, may be harmful to your health. Pulmonary emphysema and lung cancer are two startling examples of the well-known hazards of cigarette smoking.

Air pollution's major effect on health is the result of irritant materials acting on the respiratory tract. The most dangerous of these pollutants are the sulfur dioxides, nitrogen dioxide, and ozone.

These irritants have an adverse effect on the respiratory tract through a variety of mechanisms. They can cause a slowing down or stoppage of the action of the cilia in the trachea. These cilia act to propel the mucus and the particles caught in it out of the respiratory tract. The loss of this action by the cilia leaves the sensitive tissues of the lining without adequate protection. The irritants can also cause an increased production of mucus, a constriction of airways, a swelling or excessive growth of the cells that form the lining of the airways, and a change in the chemical activity of cells in the respiratory tract.

A number of epidemiological studies present solid evidence of a link between air pollution and respiratory disease. There are numerous instances where individuals, particularly those with asthma, have suffered severely from high concentrations of pollutants in the air. An increased rate of premature deaths of persons with respiratory difficulties has been associated with increased levels of air pollution.

The interpretation of health reactions to pollution depends on evidence obtained from two types of studies: toxicological and epidemiological studies. Epidemiological studies are concerned with the effects of air pollution on human populations exposed under natural conditions. Experimental studies on man and other animals where the conditions of exposure are established by the researcher fall under the category of toxicological studies.

Air pollutants exist in the solid, liquid, and gas states. The solid and liquid matter are known as particulates. Particulate size is an important factor relative to air pollutants. Particles of less than 1 micron in size are small enough to become "permanently" suspended in the air. These particles are generally referred to as aerosols. Coarse dust particles larger than 10 microns settle out of the air quickly and therefore are usually a "local" problem. Particles between 1 and 10 microns in size are capable of traveling great distances, depending on their size and wind conditions.

One of the major problems of research relative to air pollution is the constant "mix" that occurs between pollutants. Chemical activity continually occurs between particles and other substances in the air, resulting in some unexpected combinations. Small particles (less than 1 micron) can act as nuclei on which vapor condenses relatively easily. Fogs and ground mist may be so effected. Some of these particles reach deep into the lungs and can carry sulfur dioxide with them. Normally, sulfur dioxide alone would be dissolved on the mucous membrane before it reached this vulnerable tissue. These particulates may also act as catalysts. An example of this characteristic is the change of sulfur dioxide to sulfuric acid, helped on by catalytic iron oxides.

The *sources of air pollution* are divided into five categories: transportation, industry, utilities, heating, and waste disposal. The following chart presents an overview of the amount of pollutants produced in each category.

NATIONAL SOURCES OF MAJOR AIR POLLUTANTS

(millions of tons per year)

Source	Carbon Mon-oxide	Sulfur Oxides	Hydro-carbons	Nitrogen Oxides	Partic-ulate Matter	Misc. Other	Total
Transportation	66	1	12	6	1	*	86
Industry	2	9	4	2	6	2	25
Power plants	1	12	*	3	3	*	20
Space heating	2	3	1	1	1	*	8
Refuse disposal	1	*	1	*	1	*	4
Total	72	25	18	12	12	4	143

*less than 1

Transportation is the major contributor to air pollution, primarily due to the automobile. The gas powered automobile has been a hazard both in terms of fuel consumption and pollution emission.

If one measures transportation fuel consumption in BTU (British Thermal Units), the following statistics emerge:

METHOD OF TRANSPORTATION	NO. OF BTU'S PER PASSENGER MILE
Automobile	8,100 (urban) 3,400 (open highway)
Bus	3,700 (urban) 1,600 (open highway)
Train	2,900 (intercity runs)
Airplane	8,400 (large commercial aircraft)

Considering these figures one can easily conclude that bus and train travel make the most sense both in terms of fuel consumption and pollution emissions. Yet no serious effort, except perhaps indirectly through the higher costs of fuel, has been made to reduce the use of the automobile or commercial airplane as a regular means of transportation.

When sulfur-containing fuels such as oil and coal are burned, the sulfur joins with the oxygen of the air, and gaseous oxides of sulfur are the resulting by-products. Fuel combustion is the major source of the polluting oxides. Well over 36 million tons of sulfur oxides are emitted annually through the following processes:

	Million tons	%
Power Plants	20.0	55
Other Combustion	8.2	22
(Home heating and other factors)		
Smelters	4.0	11
Refineries	2.4	7
Miscellaneous	2.0	5
Total	36.6	100

If not controlled, it is estimated that sulfur oxides emission will nearly quadruple by the turn of the century.

The major oxide of sulfur that is produced in combustion is sulfur dioxide (SO_2), a colorless gas. Sulfur dioxide in turn combines easily with water vapor to become sulfurous acid (H_2SO_3), a colorless liquid. Sulfurous acid joins easily with oxygen in the air to become an extremely irritating mist known as sulfuric acid (H_2SO_4).

The sulfur oxides can affect man's breathing. When carried on particulate matter, it can cause injury to lung tissue. At sufficiently high concentrations, sulfur dioxide can cause extreme irritation to tissues of the upper respiratory tract.

Nitric oxide (NO) is formed when combustion takes place at a high enough temperature to cause a reaction between the nitrogen and oxygen of the air. Such temperatures are reached only in efficient combustion processes such as automobile cylinders, electric power plants, and other large energy-conversion processes.

Nitric oxide can be converted to nitrogen dioxide (NO_2), which is a more poisonous gas. Nitrogen dioxide is a product or by-product of numerous industries, including fertilizer and explosives manufacturing.

Exposure to high concentrations of nitrogen oxides may be fatal; however, such concentrations are highly unlikely. Prolonged exposure at ordinary concentrations may be harmful to lung tissue, the extent of which is still unknown.

Cigarette smoking has emerged as one of the major sources of "indoor" air pollution. Apart from the well-known dangers of the inhalation of tobacco smoke by smokers themselves, non-smokers may be exposed to significant air pollution from tobacco smoke in smoke-filled rooms. Carbon monoxide (CO) concentrations in rooms filled with tobacco smoke may attain or even exceed the permissible limit for occupational exposure as well as general conditions. Such concentrations are harmful to health, particularly in the case of persons already suffering from chronic bronchopulmonary and coronary heart disease.

Another possible air pollutant is ozone which is the early and continuing product of photochemical smog reaction. This reaction is brought about by the radiant energy of the sun acting upon various polluting substances. The products are known as photochemical smog. Ozone is an allotropic (one of the two or more forms of an element differing in either physical, chemical, or both properties). A molecule of ozone consists of three atoms of oxygen instead of two as in ordinary oxygen. Exposure to ozone may cause headache, severe fatigue, or coughing.

Lead (Pb) is a metallic element. As an air pollutant, lead is present in the form of particles so small that as much as 50% of what is inhaled is retained. Lead is a pollutant that is the result of the smelting process and some spraying. The major source of lead pollution, however, is the result of gasoline combustion in automobiles.

Lead in gasoline adds to the automotive pollution problem in two ways. First, lead fouls some of the major emission control systems now being developed to meet the air quality standards. Second, lead itself is a pollutant. Over 95% of the total lead emitted into the atmosphere comes from additives in gasoline.

Lead particles do penetrate the lungs and can be absorbed and retained in the blood. How much this has contributed to lead poisoning is still not clear; however, there is ample reason for concern.

Asbestos is a mineral compound used in brake linings, roofing, and insulation; in such use, asbestos dust is released into the environment. Asbestos particles have been associated with a number of lung disorders including cancer.

Hydrocarbons are compounds containing carbon and hydrocarbon. They are found in petroleum, natural gas, and coal. Most of these compounds appear harmful only in high concentrations, although research results in this area are still in an early stage.

A wide range of airborne materials known as aeroallergens is capable of eliciting a hypersensitive (allergic) response in susceptible individuals. Molds, spores, and most importantly, pollens are some of the materials known to produce such reactions. Seasonal allergic reactions first provided dramatic evidence that certain health effects may be related to specific air pollutants.

Surveys have shown that as much as 10 to 15% of the general public in some areas are allergic to what is perhaps the most common aeroallergen, ragweed pollen.[6] This allergy is commonly known as hay fever.

Precise knowledge of pollen and spore concentrations provide an indispensable aid in the diagnosis and treatment of inhalent allergy. Additional factors, including physical properties of ambient air as well as its content of inert substances, may ultimately be shown to affect respiratory responses.

WATER POLLUTION

Water is a basic requirement of life. In theory man can exist on quantities of water as small as 5 quarts a day. However, 40 to 60 quarts a day are required for our personal and domestic hygiene, if we are to remain healthy. In industrialized countries, it is not uncommon for 600 to 700 quarts to be needed per person. Such needs are becoming increasingly difficult to meet, since pollution has reduced the quality of water resources.

It is true that there is no less water on the earth than there has been in the past. However, the question of its distribution and quality has become of paramount importance.

Water is considered polluted when it is altered in composition or condition so that it is unsuitable for its intended use or purpose. Water may be considered polluted when it becomes overburdened with any of the following: infectious disease-producing agents, organic wastes, plant nutrients, inorganic chemicals, organic chemicals, sediments, radiation, thermal factors, and surface run-off.

Pollution may be accidental but is most often caused by the uncontrolled disposal of sewage and other wastes resulting from domestic and industrial processes.

Water, as part of the human environment, occurs in four forms: groundwater, fresh water masses, salt water masses, and as a vapor in the atmosphere.

Human health may be affected by ingesting water directly or in food, as well as by its use for personal hygiene, agriculture, or recreation. There are two main categories of water-related health hazards: (1) biological agents and (2) chemical and radioactive pollutants.

The biological agents transmitted in water are pathogenic bacteria, viruses, parasites, and other organisms.

The pathogenic bacteria of importance in sewage originate generally in the intestinal tract of human beings and other animals and reach the sewage by means of body discharges. Included among the pathogenic bacteria are certain specific types which, during their growth within the body of the host, produce toxic or poisonous compounds that may cause disease in the host. They may be present in sewage receiving the body discharges of persons ill with such diseases as typhoid fever, dysentery, cholera, or other intestinal infections. The possible presence of these microorganisms in sewage is one of the principal reasons why sewage must be carefully collected, adequately treated, and disposed of safely; the transfer of any sewage flows of these pathogenic or disease-producing bacteria from one person to another thus is prevented.

To determine if water is safe or if precautionary methods (chlorination) are eliminating waste, and thus pathogenic bacteria from water, it is necessary that some means be devised for detecting the number of bacteria in water. To actually detect such pathogenic bacteria as those causing typhoid fever, dysentery, or other water borne diseases is a laborious, time-consuming process. Contrary to common opinion, such examinations of water are not usually made. Rather, it is important to determine whether polluting material in the form of waste products from living animals has entered the water and to prevent further contamination from this means, or to remove the bacteria from water which has already received this type of polluting material. The procedure used is to determine the presence of an organism indicating the contamination of a water supply by the waste products from the intestinal discharges of warm-blooded animals.

All warm-blooded animals harbor parasitic bacteria of various types in their intestinal tract. These coliform bacteria are not normally pathogenic and function in the digestive processes of the host organism. They are discharged from the intestinal tract in tremendous numbers. They are present in large numbers in sewage, i.e., usually 4,000,000 to 5,000,000 coliform bacteria per ml.

If fecal discharge enters a water supply, the bacteria are carried with it and will survive there for long periods of time. Thus, their presence in a water supply provides positive evidence of pollution and the *possible* presence of the pathogenic bacteria.

The number of these coliform bacteria present can be interpreted as a measure of the safety of the water for human consumption. If large numbers of these bacteria are present, the water must be considered unsatisfactory and potentially unsafe. A simple test of water for the presence of coliform bacteria can be performed. If the laboratory tests show a concentration of coliform bacteria of less than 1 part per 100 ml. of water, the water may be considered of safe quality.

While viruses do not play a significant part in the sewage treatment process (they remain unaffected in the process), they are important since they, like pathogenic bacteria, are the causative agents of a number of diseases in man. The viruses most commonly present in polluted waters and sewage are the enteroviruses, adenoviruses, reno-viruses, and the virus (not yet identified) of infectious hepatitis. Of the enteroviruses, the spread of polio virus by water has rarely if ever been demonstrated, because of the extremely high dilution of the virus and the consequent difficulty of isolating it.

Although the virus of infectious hepatitis has not yet been isolated and identified, there is ample epidemiological evidence that outbreaks of this infection, which has a global distribution, are caused by polluted waters. The most striking example was the epidemic of infectious hepatitis in Delhi in 1955-1956, in which more than 28,000 cases were identified. Infectious hepatitis can also be spread by shellfish contamination with sewage effluent.

If present above a certain level, some chemical pollutants such as nitrates, arsenic, and lead may constitute a direct toxic hazard when ingested in water. Other water constituents, such as fluorides and chlorine, are beneficial and essential to human health if present in small concentrations, and toxic if taken in larger amounts. Recently, there has been a growing concern relative to the possible relationship of the chlorine added to drinking water (to kill bacteria) to various forms of cancer.

The consumption of water with a high nitrate concentration in infants may result in methemoglobinemia. The mean nitrate content of water consumed by affected children in Czechoslovakia ranged from 18 to 257 mg./liter, but about three-quarters of them had consumed water containing more than 100 mg./liter of nitrate.[8]

Recent research from several countries has shown an inverse statistical association between the hardness of drinkable water and the death rate from cardiovascular diseases. Areas supplied with soft drinkable water almost consistently experience a significantly higher prevalence of either arteriosclerotic heart disease, or degenerative heart disease and hypertension. One should *not* conclude from this evidence that soft water has harmful effects in human cardiovascular diseases. There is no evidence that soft water is harmful to these vascular conditions. It may be that hard water functions in a "protective" role relative to cardiovascular conditions.

NOISE POLLUTION

Noise is unwanted sound. The human ear is subject to tissue damage if exposed to sound of more than 85 decibels on the A scale for a prolonged period of time.

The effects of noise on human health range from increasing nervous tension to the actual damage of tissue in the ear. Other effects on the human system are the paling of the skin, tensing of muscles, added secretion of adrenal hormones, and increased blood pressure.

Hearing-loss problems are especially severe in certain industrial settings such as metal products production, heavy construction, motor vehicles production, and other similar industries. Recently the "acid rock musician" has been added to this list.

As stated, prolonged exposures to noise are known to lead to a gradual deterioration of the inner ear and to subsequent deafness. This occurs in addition to the normal loss of hearing that accompanies aging, referred to as presbycusis. Both presbycusis or noise induced deafness usually begin at the higher frequencies of sound. As hearing loss continues, lower frequencies also become more and more difficult to hear.

NOISE LEVELS IN DECIBELS.

Jet takeoff (nearby)	150	Threshold of pain
Hydraulic press	130	
Automobile horn		Maximum vocal effort possible
Construction noise	110	
Shout	100	
Subway station or train		Annoying
Inside car in city traffic		Limit for industrial exposures
Noisy office with machines	80	Annoying
Freeway traffic	70	Telephone use difficult
Conversation		Intrusive
Accounting Office	60	
Private business office	50	Quiet
Living room in house		
Bedroom in house	40	
Library		
Soft whisper	30	Quiet
Broadcast studio	20	
Rustling leaves in breeze	10	Barely audible

RADIATION

Radiation is a form of energy transport, while the process of radioactivity describes the nuclei of certain specific elements undergoing spontaneous disintegration and as a consequence liberating energy in the form of alpha, beta, or gamma particles.

Radioactivity, a natural phenomena, has been harnessed by man as a source of energy and a tool of medicine. Cosmic radiation has presented man with health problems relative to a number of suspected disorders. The American Medical Association has indicated its grave concern over the potential hazards to human health from over-exposure to the sun's rays, especially from sunbathing. Skin cancer and lupus are two human disorders that appear to have a direct relationship with over-exposure to the sun's rays.

The danger of radiation to human health is the result of particles penetrating human tissue and producing chemical or physical changes in the cell. No matter what the source, the sun's rays or a "leaking" nuclear device or exposure to therapeutic x ray, the danger lies in the potential effect of this exposure on human tissue. The greater the exposure, the greater the danger.

From a biological point of view, radiation effects are classified as genetic or somatic. Somatic effects produce consequences on the functioning tissue of the person exposed to radiation. Genetic effects are those which produce consequences on the chromosomes or genes in the sex cells.

EFFECTS OF SINGLE-DOSE, WHOLE-BODY RADIATION EXPOSURES IN MAN

Less than 25 rads	No observable effect
About 25 rads	Threshold level for detectable effect
About 50 rads	Slight temporary blood changes
About 100 rads	Nausea, fatigue, vomiting
200 to 250 rads	Fatality possible, though recovery is more likely
About 500 rads	Perhaps half the victims would die
About 1000 rads	All the victims would die

Artificially produced radioisotopes are used as a medical tool in both diagnosis and treatment. The progress of these radioactive drugs can be traced in the body, thus enabling the physician to measure blood flow, study the functioning of the digestive system or a specific organ, or carry out other diagnostic procedures. Radioisotopes can suppress the activity of certain tissue or destroy tissue, and often more selectively than the x-ray radiations used in cancer therapy.

PESTICIDES

The use of chemical pesticides contributes greatly toward the increase in agricultural productivity and serves as an important factor in the control of disease vectors. In using these pesticides as an instrument to control environmental conditions, man has also established a risk of uncertain magnitude. Man is thus faced with the concern of avoiding the potential dangers in the use of pesticides, while benefiting from its positive aspects.

There are four major areas of concern relative to the use of pesticides: (1) The ability of pesticides to appear far from the place of initial application; (2) the ability of some pesticides to persist and accumulate in food chains; (3) misuse in the application of pesticides; and (4) the lack of sufficient information as to the potential risks to man and other animals in the continued use of pesticides.

The primary hazard to man resulting from the use of pesticides is that of acute poisoning. The various chemicals in use as pesticides are all to some degree poisonous to some biological systems. Pesticides may enter the body through contact with the skin, through the respiratory system, and through ingestion.

Man must continue to use pesticides in agriculture and the control of disease vectors; however, he must do so with every conceivable precaution. The indiscriminate or careless use of pesticides is a condition we cannot afford.

DESIGNS FOR ACTION

In this chapter we have briefly reviewed a number of environmental health problems. It should be obvious that we stand at the center of these problems as both the victim and the culprit. From this unique and uncomfortable position, we must fight the battle against environmental pollution. What can you do now?

1. *Control the size of your family.* Limit your children to two. If a large family is desired, consider the adoption of additional children.

We tend to think that population control is the sole responsibility of the underdeveloped countries. We overlook the fact that we Americans are living in the most affluent society ever known, and that we demand more products and cause more pollution than any other country in the world. Thus, our concern for population control must become a basic priority. (See also Chapter 3 on Appreciating Sexuality.)

2. *Keep well informed.* Elect an appropriate college course to learn more about the basic principles and issues concerning environmental problems. Keep up to date on what's going on by reading *Newsweek, Time, U.S. News and World Report, The Christian Science Monitor, The New York Times,* and other magazines and newspapers. Your state and federal governments have Environmental Protection Agencies which publish current information as do many industries through their quarterly and annual reports. Membership in such voluntary organizations as the National Wildlife Federation, National Audubon Society and Sierra Club will enable you to enhance your environmental concerns and thinking.

As the Ehrlichs point out, no one knows enough to chart the future with precision. You must evaluate suggestions carefully, listen to others, compare and contrast ideas, and make your own decisions.[3]

3. *Clean up your own act.* Acquaint yourself with antipollution ordinances and abide by them. In situations where enforcement is difficult, help state and local authorities by reporting violations.

Don't be an energy hog. Keep your thermostat down to 68° in cold weather and your air conditioner up to 80° when it's hot. Buy an efficient car and keep it in good condition. Join a car pool. Use the mass transit system or ride a bike when possible.

Don't smoke and don't litter. Buy products that disintegrate or can be recycled. Use insecticides and herbicides sparingly.

By reforming your own habits to reduce pollution, you set an example for your peers to follow and become a potent force in changing lifestyles. If we really care about our water, land, and air and use a little forethought and common sense, much of this needless waste can be eliminated.[5]

4. *Join an environmentally active group* on campus or in your community. Aroused citizens concerned about the quality of the environment can both challenge and demand action by government and industry. Such a group can be composed of engineers, doctors, professors, public health officials, health educators, housewives, school personnel, business men and women, city workers, and students.

Citizen groups can be effective in demanding better sanitation, sewage treatment, water treatment, and waste disposal facilities. They can also initiate and promote action in support of recycling centers. The building of nuclear power plants and offshore oil wells has been halted by citizens groups that felt such industrial plants constituted a threat to their communities.

Such concerned groups are critically important elements in environmental movements and can carry on three fundamental missions in pursuit of a better environment:

1. to ensure that there are adequate environmental protection laws—at the community, state and federal levels—and that there are adequate appropriations and staff to carry out those laws;
2. to support, encourage and stimulate control agencies and polluters to move steadily and speedily toward compliance with environmental laws and regulations;
3. to keep the public informed, on a continuing basis, of the success—or failure—of environmental protection programs and on what still remains to be done.[10]

Pollution knows no political boundaries. You can be most successful working with a group at the community level. But what happens to your future may depend on what goes on in Washington and the United Nations, so do not be reluctant to bombard your senators and representatives with demands for appropriate action at the state, federal, and international levels. Help solve the problems rather than being a part of them!

PROBLEMS FOR YOUR CONSIDERATION

1. What are some of the psychological and social problems in this country regarding population control?

2. How have citizens' groups been effective in preventing pollution or destruction of wildlife areas?

3. Research the pros and cons of building nuclear power plants or offshore oil wells.

4. Survey your campus or local community to discover the sources and types of any pollution problems. What is being or can be done about them?

5. Review the vital statistics in your community and identify possible relationships with environmental conditions.

REFERENCES

1. Dubos, René: *Man Adapting*. New Haven, Yale University Press, 1967.
2. Ehrlich, Paul R. and Ehrlich, Anne H.: *Population Resources, Environment: Issue in Human Ecology*. San Francisco, W. H. Freeman and Co., Publishers, 1970.
3. ____: *The End of Affluence*. New York, Ballantine Books, 1974, p. 34.

4. Marine, Gene: *America the Raped.* New York, Hawthorne Books, Inc., 1967.
5. Ohio EPA: *Eco-Tips.* Columbus, Ohio, 1973.
6. Phillips, John, Jr.: *Environmental Health: A Paradox of Progress.* Dubuque, Iowa, Wm. C. Brown Company, 1971, p. 21.
7. Pohlman, Edward: *Psychology of Birth Planning.* Cambridge, Massachusetts, Schenkman Publishing Company, Inc., 1969, p. 11.
8. Schmidt, P. and Knotek, Z.: Epidemiological Evaluation of Nitrates As Ground Water Contaminants in Czechoslovakia. Paper presented to the Sixth International Water Pollution Conference, San Francisco, 1970.
9. U.S. Department of Health, Education, and Welfare: *The Health Consequences of Smoking 1974.* Washington, D.C., U.S. Government Printing Office, 1974.
10. U.S. Environmental Protection Agency: *Don't Leave It All To the Experts.* Washington, D.C., U.S. Government Printing Office, 1972.

8

Spending Your Health Dollars

In an era of scientific medicine, it is, perhaps, not too surprising that many Americans expect cures, or at least relief, to be available for most of their health problems. Fortunately, alleviation or cure *is* available for many of our health needs, but the intelligent consumer of health products and services needs to know how to select and locate those services and how to select and use health products if he is to profit from the scientific advances of recent years.

It is easier than one might believe to obtain health products and services that have little or no value and may, in fact, do harm to the consumer. How is this possible in an era when Ralph Nader and consumer protection are familiar to almost everyone? Part of the problem is related to the fact that we live in a scientific age, and *expect* science to provide us with solutions to our problems. Part lies in the fact that the media are a strong influence in our lives. Part lies in the fact that we often want to believe what we hear and read. Part lies in the fact that we are often ignorant.

This chapter will try to provide you with a sound basis for making judgments about health products and services. We want to help you spend your health dollars wisely, so that the scientific advances of recent years can help you reach or maintain a high level of positive health.

SELECTING AND USING HEALTH PRODUCTS

Many of the health products we use today are medicines. Consumers now spend about nine billion dollars annually on them, but unfortu-

129

nately, this vast expense doesn't always buy better health. The misuse of medicines is a major part of the current drug problem in this country. This isn't to suggest that medicines have no place in our lives. Indeed, they do. Knowing when and how to use them properly is the challenge.

There are two basic types of medicines: over-the-counter (OTC) drugs and prescription (Rx) drugs. *Over-the-counter drugs* (also known as patent medicines or proprietary drugs) can be purchased at drugstores, supermarkets, discount stores, and other places without a prescription. Aspirin, laxatives, cold and cough preparations, and many other types are available. If used according to the directions on the label, they are relatively safe. *Prescription drugs* carry the symbol Rx on the label, and can be purchased only when prescribed by a physician. They are generally more powerful than over-the-counter drugs and also are more likely to cause side effects.[29]

Most of us practice at least some do-it-yourself medicine. In many instances this may be an unwise practice. . . . but how do we know? Exact guidelines are difficult to state, but if the symptoms for which we are self-medicating are unusual, severe or dramatic, persistent, or recurring, it would be wise to seek the attention of a competent physician.

When considering the use of any type of medication, there are some facts to consider. Some products (OTC and Rx) relieve symptoms but don't cure the illness. Time may be all that is needed. If symptoms persist, see a physician. All medicines affect body functioning; some persons are affected adversely by products that others can take without any problems. Some medications are unsafe when taken in combination with others; avoid multi-dosing yourself. . . . and be sure your physician is aware of all OTC and Rx drugs you may be using. Many drugs deteriorate as they get old. Their potency may change, so they could be a hazard or worthless. Find out the effective and safe time span for medicines you use.

In using any medicines there are some additional guidelines to consider:

1. Read the label or ask your physician about any side effects that might be anticipated. Nausea, drowsiness, nervousness, or other side effects might occur.

2. Be certain about the amount and timing of the dose to be taken. Before or after meals? Every two or four hours? For five days? Until the prescription is used up? Should you refill the prescription?

3. Know the name of the drug. You may want to recall it later, so write it down for future reference.

4. Keep *any* and *all* medicines in places where children can't get to

them. This might mean a locked cabinet. Inconvenient? Perhaps. It might save a child's life.

Many physicians will agree that there are some medical supplies that one should have on hand . . . while keeping in mind the potential hazards to small children.[46] These include: aspirin ("adult" and baby if there are children), diarrhea medication, antihistamines for use in an allergic episode like hives, nose drops (to be used sparingly), a cough control product, petroleum jelly, gauze compresses, tape, Band-Aids, and rectal and oral thermometers. Talk with your own physician about modifications that might be suggested to make *your* medicine supply both safe and sane.

Some Special Areas of Concern

Cough and Cold Preparations. There are many of us who have at least an annual cold. Considering the nation as a whole, it is estimated that Americans suffer between 230 and 500 million colds each year, and to ease these too common sniffles and coughs over a billion dollars are spent on OTC remedies.

Most of the cold remedies contain three major ingredients: an analgesic, usually aspirin, to reduce fever, a sympathomimetic (nasal decongestant), and one or more antihistamines to dry up the mucous membranes in the nose. If taken in the specified amounts and time periods, these products are considered generally safe, but some of the ingredients are potentially dangerous. Antihistamines may cause drowsiness or dizziness. Aspirin may cause gastric irritability or bleeding from the stomach in some persons.

Further problems may arise if the cold preparation contains a variety of other ingredients, as is often the case. Caffeine may be one of these, and it may cause some persons to be nervous and jittery. Side effects of the nasal decongestants include an increase in blood pressure and heart rate, and an increased blood sugar level—the latter potentially dangerous for the diabetic. In addition, in trying to relieve one's symptoms, we may use the medication more often or in larger doses than recommended, so the side effects of the varied ingredients multiply, and may make us feel worse, rather than better.[21]

Aspirin and some extra rest are probably as effective and perhaps much safer than many of the OTC preparations. If a fever persists and additional symptoms appear, complications may have developed, thus calling for the services of a physician.

Tension Relievers. Can't sleep? Feel tense? Had a hard day? Relax! It's easy . . . if you believe all the TV advertising. Just take one of the many OTC preparations sold to reduce tension and/or induce sleep. What you may not realize is that these products are also worth little and may be extremely dangerous.

Many of these products contain an antihistamine and drowsiness *is* a side effect, as noted previously. However, investigations by the Food and Drug Administration have revealed that the usually used antihistamine failed to hasten the onset of sleep or improve its quality and later withdrawal from the product can result in unpleasant dreams and nightmares, due to disturbance of the sleep phases. Other side effects may include restlessness, nervousness, blurring of vision, ringing in the ears, and stomach irritation, rather than the desired sleep.

Other common ingredients of these OTC products include scopolamine, bromides, and salicylamide (an analgesic). Side effects from these may include hallucinations, sleeplessness, skin rashes, dizziness, and blood disorders. Researchers believe that they may work because consumers have faith in them but the possible side effects outweigh the possible values and make these products potentially more harmful than prescription drugs used for similar purposes.[22]

So . . . if you're wide awake and can't sleep, drink some warm soup and reach over to the bedside table for something to read. If sleeplessness and tension persist, see your physician.

Cosmetic Products. We need to reemphasize an old adage: Beauty *is*, indeed, more than skin deep. Yet American women, and an increasing number of men, spend an estimated six billion dollars annually for cosmetic products that are rubbed, poured, sprinkled or sprayed on, introduced into, or applied to the body for cleansing, beautifying, promoting attractiveness, or altering the appearance. This description applies to such products as toothpaste, deodorants, perfume, baby powders and dozens of others. Aside from the financial expenditure, some of these products have been shown to be of little or no value and some are known or suspected of causing adverse reactions.

However, a "revolution" in cosmetics regulation has now arrived. As of January 1, 1976, virtually all cosmetics sold in this country now list on the label or on firmly attached tags or display cards the ingredients they contain. This should be particularly beneficial to persons who are allergic to certain ingredients. Three additional voluntary regulations should also help the Food and Drug Administration enforce the provisions of the Food, Drug and Cosmetic Act: FDA has asked cosmetic manufacturers to identify themselves to the Agency by filing name and address. Second, FDA has asked that product formulas be filed. This would include the amounts of the ingredients, not just the names. Third, FDA has asked manufacturers to file data periodically on adverse reactions reported by consumers.[17] The safety of cosmetics should be increased greatly by the use of these regulations.

In using cosmetics there are a number of facts and fallacies of which the consumer should be aware.[12]

1. Cosmetics are generally safe if used as directed. Most adverse reactions are due to allergy to a specific ingredient.
2. Cosmetic allergy may be indicated by skin rashes, dry and cracked lips, headaches, hay fever symptoms, redness and itching in particular skin areas.
3. Organic or "natural" cosmetics have no special value.
4. Rare or precious ingredients are seldom if ever included in cosmetics.
5. Vitamins included in toilet preparations are not considered to be absorbed into the body in sufficient amounts to produce beneficial results.
6. The skin is nourished by normal food consumption, and not by externally applied lotions, creams, or other substances.
7. Fingernail hardeners containing formaldehyde may be injurious to users.
8. Feminine hygiene sprays are not recommended. A number of ill effects have been reported; there is no medicinal or hygienic benefit from their use.
9. Hair cannot be restored to bald heads by use of salves, ointments, or other preparations externally applied, nor by shampoos, manipulation, or mechanical devices.
10. Shampoos containing protein derivatives or amino acids have not been shown effective in preventing or curing the problem of split ends of hair.
11. Egg, herb and balsam shampoos produce few if any lasting effects.

Eye cosmetics and their use are worthy of special consideration because of the possibility of infections that could seriously damage the eyes.[11]

1. Discontinue immediately the use of any eye product that causes irritation. If irritation persists, see a doctor.
2. Recognize that your hands contain microorganisms that, if placed in the eye, could cause infections. Wash your hands before applying cosmetics to your eyes.
3. Make sure that any instrument you place in the eye area is clean.

4. Do not allow eye cosmetics to become covered with dust or contaminated with dirt or soil. Wipe off the container with a damp cloth if visible dust or dirt is present.

5. Do not use old containers of eye cosmetics. If you haven't used the product for several months, it's better to discard it and purchase a new one.

6. Do not spit into eye cosmetics. The microorganisms in your mouth may grow in the cosmetic and subsequent application to the eye may cause infection. Boiled water can be added to products which have thickened.

7. Do not share your cosmetics. Another person's microflora in your cosmetic can be hazardous.

8. Do not store cosmetics at temperatures above 85° F. Cosmetics held for long periods in hot cars, for example, are more susceptible to deterioration of the preservative.

9. Avoid using eye cosmetics if you have an eye infection or the skin around the eye is inflamed. Wait until the area is healed.

10. Take particular care in using eye cosmetics if you have any allergies.

11. When removing eye cosmetics, be careful not to scratch the eyeball or some other sensitive area.

Used wisely, and for their intended purposes, cosmetics can enhance one's appearance. Some further guidelines for action may help make them safer.[17]

1. Follow all directions and warnings. If patch testing is suggested, do it, to find out if you might be sensitive to the product.

2. Be sure your hands are clean when you apply cosmetics. Close cosmetics bottles or jars after use so they will stay clean.

3. Use your *own* cosmetics. Don't borrow another person's infections this way.

4. When a product must be moistened before use, don't use saliva. Bacteria from the mouth may be transferred.

5. If you develop an adverse reaction, discontinue using the product, see your physician, and take the cosmetic you suspect with you.

Arthritis Remedies. There are few diseases that affect as many persons as arthritis. Although not a leading "killer", arthritis *is* a leading cause of crippling and this makes the arthritis victim particularly susceptible to claims made by a variety of arthritis remedies. Since there is no positive cure for arthritis, and its discomfort is long lasting, fraudulent products (and practitioners) have a waiting clientele.

For most people with arthritis, aspirin is the best single medicine.[9] Steady dosages, taken under medical supervision, can relieve pain and reduce inflammation. For persons who cannot take aspirin, there are several other drugs that a physician can substitute. These do not include the fraudulently promoted "special" formula medicines that are sold by would-be practitioners.

A wide variety of special products has been promoted via advertising, books, and other media, for the relief of arthritis suffering.[4] Many of these are special diets or diet supplements. Honey and vinegar in combination have been suggested; sea water has been sold for as much as $3.00 a pint, and cod liver oil and orange juice and several other foods and beverages have been recommended in certain diet sequences.

Drug products also are promoted. These include the "glorified" aspirin products (aspirin plus extra ingredients), alfalfa tablets, teas and brews, and drugs available from well-advertised arthritis clinics in Mexico, other countries, and the United States itself. The products are worthless; some may be harmful.

The copper bracelet "treatment" for arthritis, although inexpensive, and harmless of and by itself, is an example of the devices sold to arthritis victims. Some devices bear exotic sounding names: Oxydonor, Inductoscope, and Z-Ray are examples. Some of these use electric current or light rays to perform their "magic". Vibrating devices and uranium gloves or treatments are equally fraudulent.

Further sources of fraudulent remedies are the mineral spas and arthritis clinics that often advertise arthritis treatment as a specialty. Legitimate clinics and physicians don't advertise; nor do they ever claim that cures can be guaranteed.

Arthritis sufferers are many, as are their problems and discomforts, but legitimate medical practitioners can provide the best care. Early diagnosis and treatment can often prevent some of the painful crippling, and self-treatment and use of devices do nothing but delay the benefits that legitimate care could bring.[8]

SELECTING YOUR HEALTH ADVISORS

Health personnel play an important role in helping you maintain positive health and return to that level following illness. The selection of competent health advisors is one of your most important responsibilities. In earlier years your family health advisors were selected by your family. While attending college, some or all of your health needs may be taken care of by the college or university health service or by local physicians whom it recommends. Today, however, more college students are married, and they may find it necessary or advisable to seek health advisors for themselves and their children. In any event, it is likely that in the near future you will be looking for competent professionals to provide care for your health needs.

The term "doctor" is familiar to all. Unfortunately, its meaning is often confusing. Those who can properly be called "doctor" may know a great deal—or nothing at all—about your health, for their professional education may be in theology, education, veterinary medicine, dentistry, osteopathy, medicine, chiropractic, or other fields. Unfortunately, some "doctors" may be self-proclaimed, or what we refer to as *quacks*—persons who claim to have medical knowledge and skills but who are not actually qualified in this way. What kind of a "doctor" do you want when you are in need of health care or advice? Who are the different "doctors" in the health field? What training have they had? What theories of health and disease do they follow?

Physicians

Medical Doctor (M.D.). The competent and well-trained physician of today is an advisor upon whom you can depend in health or illness. He or she provides preventive medical services, such as immunizations and health examinations, and when illness does occur, he can use drugs, surgery, and other scientific techniques to restore health. In all of his work, the medical doctor uses scientific research findings to support his work in the prevention and cure of disease.

A long and demanding period of education precedes licensing as a medical doctor. The medical school candidate must have a college academic background of high quality, including, in most instances, a college degree. He then goes on to a medical school for four years of study. (A few schools now have three year programs.) There are over 100 such schools in this country; most are a part of the large state university systems throughout the country, others are a part of non-public institutions. All are schools or colleges within the structure of an accredited university.

During the early years of medical studies the program focuses on preclinical scientific studies. The latter years provide an opportunity for the student to relate theory and practice as he begins caring for patients under supervision and becoming more familiar with medical specialty areas. Successful completion of this program results in the M.D.

degree, but the educational program is not yet complete. A year of hospital internship is required, following which the physician is eligible to take state examinations for licensing, and, if successful, may then begin his medical practice.

Many of today's physicians are electing to extend their education still further, and are entering residency programs following their internships. These programs, enabling them to specialize in a particular area of medicine or surgery, may be from three to five or more years in length. After two years of practice in the specialty and examinations from the Specialty Board, the physician is now Board certified.

Many families would like to have a family physician to call on for all of the family health concerns. The general medical practitioner, whose practice is not limited to any one medical field, could be this person. The family physician might also be one who has specialized in the family practice field, a relatively new area of specialty. Many adults will want an internist, (one who has specialized in the diagnosis and non-surgical treatment of diseases of the internal organs) for their general medical care. All of these physicians will, however, refer you to additional specialists when the need arises. Some of these medical specialties (M.D.) are the following:[2]

Allergy:	Diagnosis and treatment of body reactions resulting from unusual sensitivity to foods, pollens, dusts, medicines, or other substances.
Anesthesiology:	Administration of various forms of anesthesia in operations or diagnosis.
Dermatology:	Diagnosis and treatment of diseases of the skin.
Endocrinology:	Branch of medicine dealing with disorders of the glands of internal secretion.
Family Practice:	A specialty providing comprehensive and continuing medical care to a patient and his family regardless of age.
Gastroenterology:	Diagnosis and treatment of disorders of the digestive tract.
Geriatrics:	Branch of medical practice concerned with the clinical treatment of old age and its manifestations.
Gynecology:	Diagnosis and treatment of diseases of the female reproductive organs.
Hematology:	Diagnosis and treatment of diseases of the blood and blood-forming organs.

Internal Medicine:	Diagnosis and non-surgical treatment of illnesses of adults.
Laryngology:	Diagnosis and treatment of diseases of the larynx.
Nephrology:	The practice of internal medicine as it relates to diseases of the urinary system.
Neurology:	Diagnosis and treatment of diseases of the brain, spinal cord, and nerves.
Obstetrics:	Care and treatment during pregnancy, childbirth, and postpartum period.
Ophthalmology:	Diagnosis and treatment of diseases of the eye, including prescribing glasses.
Otology:	Diagnosis and treatment of diseases of the ears.
Otorhinolaryngology:	Diagnosis and treatment of diseases of the ear, nose, and throat.
Pediatrics:	Prevention, diagnosis and treatment of children's diseases.
Psychiatry:	Diagnosis and treatment of mental disorders.
Radiology:	Use of radiant energy including x-rays, radium, cobalt 60, etc. in the diagnosis and treatment of disease.
Rhinology:	Diagnosis and treatment of diseases of the nose.
Surgery, Cardiovascular:	Diagnosis and surgical treatment of diseases of the heart and blood vessels.
Surgery, General:	Diagnosis and treatment of disease by surgical means, without limitation to special organ systems or body regions.
Surgery, Orthopedic:	Diagnosis and surgical treatment of diseases, fractures, and deformities of the bones and joints.

Doctor of Osteopathy (D.O.). Doctors of Osteopathy are trained in all branches of medicine, including the use of drugs and surgery. In addition, the osteopathic physician is trained in manipulation.

Dr. Andrew Taylor Still, the founder of osteopathy, worked out a system of manipulation intended to realign functional deviations and abnormalities. His rationale for this was a belief that the body is self healing, that its adequate functioning depends upon its unimpaired structure, and that an uninterrupted nerve and blood supply to tissues is indispensable to the normal functioning of all parts of the body.[25] Manipulation is not the only type of therapy used by the osteopathic physician. As noted earlier, he is trained in all areas of medicine, and uses drugs and surgery in treating disease. He may *also* use manipulation.

The majority of students in osteopathic colleges have received bachelor's degrees; some may have entered following three years of undergraduate preparation. During the first two years of osteopathic education, basic sciences are emphasized; the last two years of the program provide for clinical training. Following successful completion of this program, the student will intern for a year in an osteopathic hospital, take state licensing examinations, and then be eligible to practice. There are also opportunities for specialization. Residency programs are two to five years in length and certification examinations may be taken following two years of specialized practice. Areas of specialization include internal medicine, obstetrics and gynecology, pediatrics, dermatology, and a number of others. The osteopathic physician may practice in all states (if he has taken their licensing examination), but may be restricted in some states in his use of drugs and/or surgery.

At the present time there are 9 schools of osteopathic medicine in the United States. One of these is a part of a large state university system in the midwest; the others are independent institutions and are not a part of any university.

You have undoubtedly noticed that the education and licensing of the D.O. and that of the M.D. appear similar. In more recent years their programs have become more comparable, and in some states osteopathic physicians are being invited to join state medical societies and, after specified postgraduate training, to be recognized as M.D.'s. This practice is not yet widespread.

Physician's Assistants

Since approximately the mid-sixties, there have developed in this country over 200 programs to train personnel to assist physicians in providing health care.[41] This concept and the programs have arisen in response to the need for more care for more people, and the shortage of physicians, especially in rural areas.

The term, "physician's assistant," and its precise meaning are difficult to explain at this time. Some of these programs are providing advanced training for nurses to qualify them as pediatric nurse practitioners; others are training personnel to provide specific technical assistance; still others are providing training of such breadth that the assistant could perform diagnostic and therapeutic procedures specified by the physician and could work in settings apart from the physician. Programs for training these assisting personnel are of varied duration; the more extensive ones are two years in length.

A number of studies have been conducted in recent years to try to determine the satisfaction of persons who have been cared for by these assistants.[18,26] One of the main concerns appears to be indecision about the role and responsibilities of the assistant. Some persons are not yet willing to permit a non-physician to perform traditional physician duties, but there seem to be indications that at least some of these duties *can* be performed by a well-trained non-physician. Future years will undoubtedly bring more clarification of the roles of these assisting personnel.

Dentists

The dental field is considerably less complicated than the medical one. Dentists have either a *Doctor of Dental Surgery* degree (D.D.S.) or a *Doctor of Dental Medicine* degree (D.M.D.), depending upon the degree awarded by the dental school from which they graduated. In either case, they are well trained to treat tooth, jaw, and gum diseases, and to offer preventive services such as topical fluoride applications and cleanings. Before beginning his professional training the dental student has had a minimum of three years of college (usually four) and has had to demonstrate ability and aptitude for this profession.

Several of the more common dental specialists are:

Orthodontist—   a specialist in the prevention and correction of malocclusion.

Pedodontist—   a specialist in the prevention and treatment of pathologic oral conditions which occur during childhood.

Periodontist—   a specialist in the prevention and treatment of the diseases affecting the tissues which support, attach and surround the teeth.

Additional Eye Health Personnel

We have already mentioned the *ophthalmologist* (oculist), the medical specialist who treats diseases and disorders of the eyes and vision. There are also other personnel in this field:

Optometrist   one whose education, training and licensure
(O.D.)—   qualify him to examine eyes, without the use of drugs, for abnormal visual problems not due to disease. He may prescribe, fit,

and supply eyeglasses and provide visual training for such conditions. The optometrist is a graduate of a school or college of optometry and receives at least five years of study beyond the high school level. He must take a state licensing examination in order to practice. His license does not permit him to use drugs or surgery in his practice.

Optician — a skilled technician who is qualified to grind lenses, fit, and dispense eyeglasses. Some states require licensing.

Orthoptist — trained to correct strabismus and strengthen weakened eye muscles by means of exercises prescribed by an ophthalmologist. Training programs are fifteen months in length, following two years of college or comparable education.

Limited Practitioners

Practitioners of medicine and surgery are licensed to practice following successful completion of examinations given by the medical boards of the various states. Some practitioners are licensed as "limited practitioners" because their education focuses on a single therapeutic system or treatment for the relief or cure of disease, and does not involve the use of drugs or major surgery. Thus, the services they perform are limited by law, as well as by their educational background. "Limited practitioner" licensing varies somewhat from state to state. Two such practitioners are mentioned here.

Doctor of Podiatric Medicine (Pod. D.). The podiatrist (formerly known as chiropodist) is concerned with the diagnosis, prevention, and treatment of foot disorders. This doctor has received his training at a four-year college of podiatry, following at least two years of college work. There are five colleges of podiatric medicine in this country. Podiatrists must take a state examination for licensing.[6]

Doctor of Chiropractic (D.C.). Chiropractors consider their system a natural, drugless healing method, in which health is maintained by establishing a perfect alignment of the body's bone and nerve structure. This system of treatment is based on the belief that the nervous system controls all other systems and all physiological functions of the human body. When the nerve control to body systems is interfered with, function is impaired, the body is less resistant to infection or other stimuli, and disease occurs.[1]

High school graduation is the minimum requirement for admission to the chiropractic colleges, although more than half the states require at least two years of pre-chiropractic college work for licensure. The college course of study is four years.

Other Practitioners

You will occasionally become aware of several other practitioners (also limited by state laws) in the health field. Mechanotherapists, naturopaths, electrotherapists, and others use different types of treatment such as sun, electricity, mechanical devices, and water in the treatment of disease. Educational requirements and professional training in these fields are varied, but are not on a level with those in the medical field. The consumer needs to be aware of the possibility of quackery in these areas.

The Quackery Problem

There is some concern today that quack or fraudulent health practitioners *do* exist. Their areas of "specialization" may vary, but they are frequently found working in areas in which modern medicine and science have not yet been completely successful. Cancer, arthritis, and sexual problems are three of the areas where fraudulent practice may be found.

When cancer is treated early, before spreading, the cure rate is good for many types, but the fears and the failures encourage the incompetent and fraudulent to make money at the cost of lives. So-called "cancer clinics" operating in Mexico and other countries, use methods and materials that have not been proven effective and, in doing so, keep patients from receiving the care which might save their lives.[35]

Arthritis and rheumatism are other fields for exploitation. No cures are known, and sufferers number in the millions. The exploiters have their own curative products and practices and reap financial benefits of over $400,000,000 annually. The side effects of some of these treatments are worse than the diseases themselves, and don't improve or cure the original problem.[34]

Phony sex clinics capitalize upon another area of human concern. It is estimated that as many as 5000 such clinics have developed during the past few years. Their treatment proposals are often emotionally traumatic as well as unsound, and may make future, legitimate sexual counseling much more difficult.[23]

A word of caution might be said here about the women's sex clinics that have developed recently. Some, established by competent personnel, can, indeed, help women understand their unique sexuality concerns and receive gynecological care from able, caring persons. Others, promoting do-it-yourself gynecology or utilizing untrained or unethical practitioners, have the potential for great harm, and may keep women from receiving examinations and treatment from competent physicians.

Fraudulent health care can be physically and/or emotionally traumatic, and may result in death. Other health areas to watch are weight reduction, mental health counseling, and procedures designed to increase breast size. Your best defense is to have a competent, ethical physician, and to seek his advice before seeking other health care. We realize that even competently provided care is often long-term, and not always successful, but its potential for success far outweighs "care" provided by fraudulent practitioners.

How to Spot a Health Quack

Certain signals should arouse your suspicions that a medical quack is looking at your pocketbook. The Department of Investigation of the American Medical Association says to beware if:[3]

1. He uses a special or "secret" formula or machine that he claims can cure diseases.
2. He promises a quick or easy cure.
3. He advertises, using "case histories" or testimonials to impress people.
4. He clamors constantly for medical investigation and recognition.
5. He claims medical men are persecuting him or that they are afraid of his competition.
6. He tells you that his method of treatment is better than surgery, x rays, or drugs.

How to Choose Your Health Advisors

Let us suppose, now, that you have made a decision. You know what type of medical or dental care you wish to have, but you don't know how to find it. This may seem like a simple problem, but it takes consideration and is worthy of time and effort *before* the emergency or other situation that requires medical or dental care. The following suggestions might be of assistance:

1. Ask your hometown health advisors if they can recommend advisors in your new community.
2. Ask educated, alert persons who have lived in your new community long enough to have selected health advisors. Your minister or employer might be able to make suggestions.
3. Ask the local medical and dental societies for the names of several advisors whom they would recommend in your area of the community.
4. Compare the lists of names you have. Are any advisors mentioned by several sources? This may be a sign worth noting.
5. Consult the *American Medical Directory* and the *Directory of Medical Specialists*. These are available at public libraries, medical associations, and hospitals. From these you will be able to learn the physician's age, educational background, experience and professional affiliations.
6. Make an appointment to visit one or more of the physicians or dentists. In addition to professional expertise, you want health advisors who are sincere and with whom you can communicate easily. Discuss their hospital affiliations and their availability for home and night visits. If your family includes children, older persons or those with any special health problems, these special needs should be discussed.

Choose your health advisors carefully. These are among the most important decisions you will ever make.

Guidelines for Being a Better Patient

Good medical care is not the responsibility of the physician alone. We, the patients, often would receive better care if we were better patients. A physician has suggested some of these Do's and Don'ts that should help you get maximum benefit from your medical visits:[27]

1. Do—when you call the doctor's office for an appointment, tell his nurse or secretary roughly what your problem is, so that she can allow enough time for your office visit.
2. Do—organize your thoughts. An accurate history of an illness is important. How long have you had the pain? What foods, if any, produce it? Do any medicines relieve it?
3. Do—cooperate during the physical examination. Don't try

to talk the physician out of doing pelvic and rectal exams. Don't object when the physician has his nurse carry out some of the routine procedures.

4. Do—ask questions of your physician. What is the medicine he's prescribing? Why does he believe you need a certain type of surgery? What are his fees?

5. Do—follow instructions. Return for follow-up visits, take your medications as directed, stay on your diet!

and now the Don'ts:

1. Don't—if you can help it, take up more of the physician's time than was originally planned for. If you want a physical exam, be sure it's known when your appointment is made— not when he has finished treating your sore throat.

2. Don't—lie to the doctor, or yourself. Your physician wants to treat you, not judge you. Be honest about your smoking, drinking, or sexual practices, as well as about your symptoms.

3. Don't—ask for unnecessary pills. Many illnesses are minor and self-limiting. Time, rather than medication, may be the best treatment, and your physician may not feel that medication is necessary.

4. Don't—ask to be hospitalized unnecessarily. This increases hospitalization insurance rates for all.

5. Don't—leave your doctor's office dissatisfied. If you are not satisfied with what your physician has or hasn't done, talk with him about it.

Remember . . . good medical care involves a cooperative and understanding relationship between a competent physician and a responsible patient.

PAYING THE COST OF HEALTH CARE

In recent years there has developed much concern about some problems related to health care in the United States. Rather than being considered as a privilege, health care is now more often viewed as a *right* for all Americans. This concept has several implications: the quality of health care must be good; health care personnel and services must be distributed throughout the country so they are accessible to all; health care must be priced so that all can afford it. American health care is generally viewed as of high quality; its accessibility and its cost are, however, two problems.

At the present time, the responsibility of paying for health care is still largely a personal one. How can you do it? What options do you have? These are some questions you will need to consider.

Health Insurance

Health insurance is one means by which at least 80% of the population tries to protect itself from the high costs of medical care. With but few exceptions, this insurance does not, however, cover routine medical costs. It is primarily useful in helping to pay for hospital and hospital-related expenses. Many of you are still covered by your parents' health insurance policies. Some colleges and universities make available to students, through private insurance companies, policies that students may purchase. If you are a student who has a family to support, you may need or already have a policy of your own. Regardless of the source of your policy, it is helpful to understand what type of protection is available in different types of policies.

Perhaps we should discuss another question before going any further: Why should you have health insurance? Your age group is, in general, a healthy one. Why spend the money? It's true that the majority of you won't be in the hospital this year. . . . but what would happen if you *were?* Each person needs to look at his own situation when answering this question.

How would you pay a hospital bill of $1000, $2000, $5000 or $10,000? These are not uncommon expenses today. Basic costs for room, meals and usual nursing care may be as much as (or more than) $100 a day; added to this would be the costs of medications, extra nursing care, x rays, operating room charges, doctors' bills, intensive care charges, and others that accumulate when one is ill. What financial resources do you have to draw on? Could your family help? What hardships would this involve? How likely are you to be hospitalized? Children and young adults have a high accident rate; older persons are more likely to experience illnesses. Families with young children often have unexpected medical expenses. These are a few of the considerations involved when you survey your need for health insurance. Many people feel that they want health insurance even if they don't use it.

Before purchasing insurance it is necessary to decide the type of health expenses you want to be protected against and the extent of the protection you desire. There are five different categories or types of protection you might desire.

Hospital insurance provides assistance in the payment of hospital room and board charges, usual nursing care, drugs, laboratory expenses, and others. Some hospital plans provide for complete payment of all bills, (with perhaps some exceptions, such as diagnostic tests or blood plasma), while others allow up to specified amounts for certain services, and the patient pays the difference between the allowance and the actual bill.

Surgical insurance provides for the payment of all or part of the doctor's fee for an operation.

Regular medical expense insurance provides benefits for the payment of doctor's home and office visits, laboratory work, and other expenses.

Major medical or catastrophe insurance is designed to assist in the payment of heavy hospital and surgical bills—those that run into the thousands of dollars. Many of these policies are written with a deductible amount, like auto insurance, with the individual paying the first hundred dollars or five hundred dollars or whatever the deductible amount is, and the insurance company paying the remainder of the bill or 75 or 80% of it.

Loss-of-income insurance pays the individual cash benefits weekly or monthly if he is unable to work due to illness or accident.

Many college students will find health insurance plans available to them through their colleges and universities at nominal rates. This is *group insurance*, similar to that available to employee groups in industry and business. Group policies are usually less expensive than similar insurance purchased individually, and the benefits may be more extensive. Most students feel such coverage is a necessity as well as a wise purchase.

Most wise consumers are good shoppers. They know quality. Quality is also important when health insurance is purchased, and after deciding what basic type you desire, there are a number of items that can help you to determine the quality of the plans presented by different companies. First, of course, do your business with a reputable insurance company. The major, well established firms offer reliable protection. Talk to their agents and compare the coverage provided by the different companies. How many hospital days are provided for? How does the allowance for hospital room and board charges compare with the hospital rates in your area? Are drugs, x rays, special nursing services, and other expensive extra costs provided for? If you are married, are your dependents covered as fully as you are? Are maternity benefits provided? Does the "deductible" apply to each family member or to the whole family? In general, try to compare the plans, item by item, and determine which one gives you the most protection of the type you desire for the money involved. As in the purchase of other consumer goods, you generally get what you pay for.

Some persons are eligible for a federal government health insurance program administered by the Social Security Administration. (See also Chapter 9.) This program is Medicare, for people sixty-five years of age and over and some people under sixty-five who are disabled. Medicare has two parts; one is hospital insurance, the other medical insurance.

Medicare's hospital insurance will help pay for medically necessary inpatient hospital care, and after a hospital stay, for inpatient care in a skilled nursing facility and for care at home by a home health agency. There are certain limits on how many days of care and home health visits can be covered. Major services covered include a semi-private room, meals, usual nursing care, intensive care, operating room costs, drugs, x rays and others.

Medicare's medical insurance will help pay for medically necessary doctor's services, outpatient hospital services, outpatient speech pathology and physical therapy services, x rays, and some others.

Medicare is available to persons over sixty-five years of age (and under sixty-five if disabled) whether or not they have credits for work under Social Security. If they do not have such credits, they must pay separate monthly premiums for both the hospital and medical insurance. At the time of this writing, these costs would total about $43.00 a month, and could be expected to increase as hospital costs increase. Persons eligible under Social Security do not pay any premium for the hospital insurance. The medical insurance is about $7.00 a month at this time.[44]

Many persons feel that some form of national health insurance program will be enacted by Congress within the next year or two. The reasons, as expressed by Alice Rivlin,[30] are that the poor are still inadequately covered by any form of health insurance, few Americans are protected against catastrophically high medical bills, and the present health insurance system discourages preventive medicine (since it usually pays only when one is ill and hospitalized).

A variety of plans has been proposed. In general, they can be divided into two groups. The first group would involve a system in which health care insurance policies would be purchased from private insurance companies for beneficiaries by employers and/or government agencies. Programs included in the second group propose to provide health care cost coverage through the Social Security System. These latter proposals would be financed by increased Social Security payments or taxes on individuals and their employers.[20]

Many nations have preceded the United States in the development of national health care and health insurance programs. Great Britain, Canada, Sweden and Russia are some of these. Reports of success, satisfaction, dissatisfaction, abuse, and inefficiency can be found. If or when any large scale changes occur in American health insurance and health care programs, most Americans want to be assured of the availability of high quality medical care at a price they can afford to pay.

Health Care Delivery

The traditional pattern for the provision of health care in the United States is the private physician-patient one, and most Americans still seek a private practitioner for their care. In some sections of the country various types of group practices have developed, where a group of physicians, representing general and specialty medicine, join together to care for the varied health needs of patients. Most of these group practices are on a fee-for-service basis, as with one's family physician and others to whom he might refer you.

Some of the group practice plans that have developed take a different form. They not only provide the care, but also offer a prepaid comprehensive medical care program. Membership in the plan provides assurance that complete medical care, including hospitalization, will be provided to the subscriber. The Kaiser Foundation Health Plan, available in several west coast areas, and New York City's Health Insurance Plan are two well known examples.

In December, 1973, The Health Maintenance Organization Act (often referred to as HMO) became a part of federal legislation. This HMO Act is designed to stimulate the development of an alternative organizational structure for the delivery of health services. This structure is similar in concept to the prepaid medical care programs just described. The HMO Act provides financial assistance in the development of these programs and for regulation to see that they continue to meet the requirement of the law. Monies are not available to pay for the health services provided to patients. Prospective patients will join, on an annual fee basis, and then be eligible to receive the comprehensive services that are specified in the Act. These include physician services, hospital inpatient and outpatient services, emergency care, mental health care, treatment for drug or alcohol abuse, diagnostic and therapeutic radiologic services, home health visits, and preventive health services, including family planning services, infertility services, eye examinations for children, and dental care for children.

HMO coverage provides more services than many currently existing health insurance policies. Where available, they may be highly competitive if their costs are not too much more than what families or individuals are now paying for health insurance. It would be expected that "membership" in an HMO would reduce the medical costs that one normally incurs that are not now covered by insurance.[13,16] In conclusion, then, we might suggest these guidelines for action:

Survey your own need for health care and the responsibility you have for the health care of any dependents you may have.

Investigate health care costs in your community.

Consider the financial resources you have to meet expected *and* unexpected health care expenses.

Explore the health care programs available through your college or university or your employer.

Explore other health care plans available in your community.

Compare costs and benefits of all programs.

Investigate the reputation of the companies and organizations offering the programs.

Select a program that will provide for your needs and give you the most for your money.

AGENCIES THAT HELP TO PROTECT OUR HEALTH

Even the most intelligent consumer needs the additional protection offered by several government agencies. Particularly noteworthy are the activities of these: the Food and Drug Administration, the Federal Trade Commission, and the Post Office Department.

The Food and Drug Administration. FDA carries out the responsibilities assigned to it by the Congress. Four laws authorize the majority of FDA activities:[45]

1. The Federal Food, Drug and Cosmetic Act requires that foods be safe and wholesome, that drugs be safe and effective, and that cosmetics and medical devices be safe. All these products must be properly labeled.

2. The Fair Packaging and Labeling Act requires that labeling be honest and informative, so that shoppers may easily determine the best value.

3. The Radiation Control for Health and Safety Act protects consumers from unnecessary exposure to radiation from x-ray machines and consumer products such as microwave ovens and color TVs.
4. The Public Health Service Act establishes FDA's authority over vaccines, serums and other biological products. It also is the basis for FDA's programs on milk sanitation, shellfish sanitation, restaurant operations and interstate travel facilities.

Some of the activities performed by the FDA include the following: inspecting plants where foods, drugs, cosmetics or other products are made or stored, to make sure good practices are being observed; reviewing and approving new drug applications and food additive petitions before they can be used; approving every batch of insulin and antibiotics and most color additives, before they can be used; setting standards and testing consumer products, such as foods that are made according to a set recipe (such as peanut butter); conducting reviews of all prescription and non-prescription medicines, biological drugs, and veterinary products now on the market.

In addition the agency develops regulations for proper labeling, helps industries it regulates to develop better quality control, tests drugs after approval to be sure they meet standards, and issues warnings to the public when hazardous products have been identified.

Although the FDA *can* do many things to help the consumer, there are some misconceptions about its legal authority. It cannot prevent a person from selling products such as worthless medical devices or harmful cosmetics until they are actually marketed—FDA has to prove they are worthless or harmful; it can generally act only against products sold in interstate commerce; it cannot recall a product without legal action; it can't control product prices; it can't directly regulate the advertising of any product except prescription drugs. FDA *can* and *does* go to court to seize illegal products and to prosecute the manufacturer, packer, or shipper of adulturated or mislabeled products.[45]

Within the last two years the Supreme Court has supported (against drug company lawsuits) FDA's right to require scientific proof of drug effectiveness, and endorsed the agency's mass review of the safety, effectiveness, and labeling of all over-the-counter drugs. This review is currently underway. Additional reviews will include biological drugs, therapeutic devices, diagnostic products, and "generally recognized as safe" food additives.

As consumers, we are aware of the results of some recent FDA actions. Botulism-contaminated mushrooms were withdrawn from the market, blood banking and processing establishments are being inspected, ingredient labeling for cosmetics became effective January 1, 1976, and radiation safety for patients will be increased because of new protection features in diagnostic equipment. In addition, hundreds of unsafe toys were recalled during a recent year and over 1500 drug recalls took place.[19] One of FDA's older but never-to-be-forgotten actions was in 1962 when it refused to permit the sale of thalidomide, because of inadequate testing by the manufacturer. Thalidomide was manufactured and sold abroad, however, and many children and families are living with the severe birth defects it caused.

The FDA has more than 100 offices across the United States, so many Americans can easily reach them. If we find a product regulated by FDA that appears to be mislabeled, unsanitary, harmful, or in violation of the law, we should call or write to them. We should note, too, that our own intelligent selection and use of products is crucial, if we are to be as well protected as we desire.

The Federal Trade Commission. The Federal Trade Commission is charged with keeping competition both free and fair. In doing this it attempts to safeguard the consuming public by preventing the dissemination of false or deceptive advertisements of foods, drugs, cosmetics, therapeutic devices, and other unfair or deceptive practices. In addition, it regulates packaging and labeling of certain consumer commodities so as to prevent consumer deception and facilitate value comparison.[42]

Recent activities of this agency have included the restricting of misleading advertising associated with vitamin and food supplement plans and restrictions against books advertising cures for a wide variety of ills.

The Post Office Department. Existing laws permit the Post Office Department to take action against quacks who use the mails in an attempt to bilk the public in a "false or fraudulent" manner. Notices of such postal seizures appear regularly in the FDA Consumer, a publication written especially for the public. In recent months these have included products for treating skin disorders, wrinkle removers, baldness cures, weight control products, smoking deterrents, and sex stimulants.[36-39]

THE CONSUMER'S CHOICE

Being alert to the possibility of fraud and deception in the area of health products and services is one of the best ways to avoid being deceived. You can protect your health *and* your pocketbook if you will give consideration to the following recommendations when spending your dollars:

1. Rely on the advice of your physician when considering the purchase of specific products that claim health benefits.
2. Avoid the purchasing of special health foods, food supplements, and vitamins, unless they are prescribed by your physician. A well-balanced diet will take care of your nutritional needs.
3. Learn to recognize the various "pitches" of the modern medicine man.
4. Be suspicious of health products sold by door-to-door salesmen.
5. Be wary of all products and mechanical devices that are claimed to be useful for the cure of arthritis, rheumatism, cancer, and other chronic diseases.
6. Be alert when reading advertisements for health products.
7. Look for proprietary drug products (nonprescription drugs) that bear the letters U.S.P. or N.F., meaning that they meet the standards of identity, purity, and strength established by the United States Pharmacopeia or National Formulary.
8. Read the labels on the products you purchase. The Food, Drug and Cosmetic Act requires that the label tell contents, what the product will do, how to use the product, and any cautions that should be observed in its use.
9. Do not hesitate to contact the Better Business Bureau, local Medical Society, Food and Drug Administration offices, or the Post Office Department if you believe you have discovered a fraudulent product or scheme.

Professional Organizations

The varied and widespread problems of consumer health are also of concern to a number of professional organizations. The American Medical Association, the American Dental Association, and the Better Business Bureau are several of these groups that are interested in helping their own members and the consumer become better informed about the products and services that they use.

The *American Medical Association's* Department of Investigation has the largest file in existence on medical quackery, and cooperates with law enforcement agencies by providing evidence leading to convictions. Other departments and committees of the Association are similarly engaged in trying to provide for the better health of the American people. Publications of the *American Dental Association* include materials on the care of the teeth, fluoridation, diet and dental health, and various pamphlets for parents and teachers. An extensive film collection, available on a rental basis, also aids in educating the school child and the citizen about the benefits of adequate and reliable dental care. The *Better Business Bureau* keeps its members (business and professional firms and their employees) informed about questionable business practices in the community by means of special bulletins, and investigates and acts upon complaints of unfair and unethical business practices. The Bureau provides a valuable public service through its many activities against unscrupulous advertising, misleading promotion schemes, and the distribution of fraudulent and worthless "cures."

What Can The Consumer Do?

There are few college students or their professors who have money to throw away, yet that is what they and many other Americans are doing daily, as they spend money and risk their lives by using worthless products and fraudulent medical care. The total bill is at least a billion dollars a year, a sum that well might be put to better use. The human cost cannot be estimated.

What factors are involved in this unnecessary waste of lives and money? *Ignorance* is undoubtedly involved in some instances. Many people do not know how to avoid a quack practitioner, do not know that at the present time diabetes can be controlled but not cured, do not know that all cancer *isn't* hopeless if it receives proper and early medical care. The college student who continues to keep up with health and medical developments should be able to protect himself from fraudulent schemes.

Equally as dangerous as ignorance is *apathy*, a second factor that retards health progress. The college students who use tranquilizers and/or amphetamine ("keep awake") pills; the person who knows the dangers of self-medication, but continues to use lozenges, cough medicines, and other products to treat his illnesses; these are the apathetic members of our population—the ones with the "So what?" or "Who cares?" attitude.

Fear is one of the greatest problems in this area of frauds and quackery. Fear of doctors and hospitals, surgery, medical examination, and other procedures may lead persons to use products and services that assure them of cures without surgery, hospitalization, or any of the truly miraculous procedures that can bring health and better living to those who avail themselves of them at an early stage of their illnesses.

If you have a broad background of information and understanding in the health field and know where to seek reliable information, you are in a position to be able to avoid the frauds and quackery that appear on the American scene. Knowledge will decrease any normal fears you may have and help you make judgments based on scientific information, rather than on the basis of hearsay, advertising, or the clever patter of a talented but misleading salesman.

For better living and positive health, consider these designs for action:

Evaluate advertisements carefully. . . .

Choose health advisors in relation to their scientific training and philosophies. . . .

Report suspected frauds to appropriate authorities. . . .

Let your local, state, and national representatives know that you want them to support legislation designed to combat frauds. . . .

BE AN INTELLIGENT CONSUMER!!!!

PROBLEMS FOR YOUR CONSIDERATION

1. Compare the provisions of several different hospitalization insurance policies. How do they differ? Is any one apparently a better buy than the others for you at this time?

2. What health services are available to you through your college or university student health service? For which ones are extra fees (beyond your student health fee) charged? Are any services available to your dependents? Does your school make available, perhaps for an extra fee, any hospital or medical insurance for you and/or your dependents? How inclusive are the benefits?

3. Investigate the licensing procedures in your state for selected medical and health personnel. What educational requirements must they meet? What sorts of examinations must they take? What kinds of health care do their licenses permit them to provide? How often do their licenses have to be renewed?

4. Look up articles in *Consumer Reports* and *Consumer's Research* on some over-the-counter drugs or cosmetic products. On what basis are the products compared? Are any of the products in the same category judged to be a better buy than the others? Why?

5. Does your medicine cabinet contain any prescription products that were left over from the illness for which they were prescribed? Check with a pharmacist to find out which ones should be discarded to avoid the possible risks of deterioration.

REFERENCES

1. American Chiropractic Association: *Planning a Career in Chiropractic.* Des Moines, The Association, n.d.
2. American Medical Association, Department of Health Education: Correspondence with Dr. Wallace A. Wesley, Director, January, 1975.
3. _____: *Facts About Quacks.* Chicago, The Association, 1971, p. 2.
4. _____: *Health Quackery–Arthritis.* Chicago, The Association, 1968.
5. American Osteopathic Association: *The Profession of Osteopathic Medicine.* Chicago, The Association, n.d.
6. American Podiatry Association: *Doctor of Podiatric Medicine: Partner for Health.* Washington, The Association, n.d.
7. American Public Health Association: Health Maintenance Organizations: A Policy Paper, *American Journal of Public Health*, 61: (December, 1971).
8. The Arthritis Foundation, New York, N.Y. Correspondence, January, 1975.
9. _____: *The Truth About Aspirin for Arthritis.* New York, The Foundation, 1970.
10. Behind FDA's Regulations, *FDA Consumer*, 8: (December, 1974—January, 1975).
11. Bruch, Carl W.: Eye Products: Handle With Care. *FDA Consumer*, 6: (July-Aug., 1972).
12. Cosmetics and Personal Grooming Aids, *Consumer's Research*, 10: (October, 1974).
13. Dorsey, Joseph L.: The Health Maintenance Organization Act of 1973 (P.L. 93-222) and Prepaid Group Practice Plans, *Medical Care*, 13: (January, 1975).
14. *Education Annual, 1974:* A Supplement to Vol. 73 of the *Journal of the American Osteopathic Association.*
15. Fuller, John G.: *200,000,000 Guinea Pigs.* New York, G. P. Putnam's Sons, 1972.
16. HMO Legislation Directed Toward More Benefits for More People, *Geriatrics*, 29: (July, 1974).
17. Heenan, Jane: A Revolution in Cosmetics Regulation, *FDA Consumer*, 8:16, (April, 1974).
18. Henriques, Charles, *et al.*: Performance of Adult Health Appraisal Examinations Utilizing Nurse-Practitioners-Physician Teams and Paramedical Personnel. *American Journal of Public Health*, 64: (Jan., 1974).
19. Janssen, Wallace F.: 1973: Reflecting A New Perspective, *FDA Consumer*, 8: (April, 1973).
20. Jonas, Steven: Issues in National Health Insurance in the United States of America, *The Lancet*, 2: (July 20, 1974).
21. Katz, Sol: Evaluating the Cold Remedies, *Today's Health*, 52: (February, 1974).
22. Mark, Norman: Calm Down—At Your Own Risk, *Today's Health*, 52: (March, 1974).
23. Masters, William H. with Max Gunther: Phony Sex Clinics—Medicine's Newest Nightmare, *Today's Health*, 52: (November, 1974).

24. Michaelson, Mike: How Your Man Can Crown Himself With Glory . . . When His Hairline Starts Retreating, *Today's Health*, 51: (March, 1973).
25. Mills, Lawrence W.: *The Osteopathic Profession and its Colleges*. Chicago, American Osteopathic Association, n.d., p. 3.
26. Nelson, Eugene C., Jacobs, Arthur and Johnson, Kenneth: Patients' Acceptance of Physician's Assistants. *Journal of the American Medical Association*, 228: (April 1, 1974).
27. Nolen, William: Rules to Make You A Better Patient, *Today's Health*, 51: (April, 1973).
28. Palmer, Beverly B.: A Model for a Community-Based Women's Clinic, *American Journal of Public Health*, 64: (July, 1974).
29. A Primer on Medicines, *FDA Consumer*, 8: (December, 1973-January, 1974).
30. Rivlin, Alice: Agreed: Here Comes National Health Insurance. Question: What Kind? *The New York Times Magazine*, Section 6: (July 21, 1974).
31. Roemer, Milton and Shonick, William: HMO Performance: The Recent Evidence, *Milbank Memorial Fund Quarterly*. 51: (Summer, 1973).
32. Rosen, Samuel: Beware of the 'Quackupuncturist' Who Operates for Profit, *Today's Health*, 52: (August, 1974).
33. Schaller, Warren E. and Carroll, Charles R.: *Health Quackery and the Consumer*. Philadelphia, W. B. Saunders Co., 1976.
34. Schultz, Terri, with Bard Lindeman: The Pain Exploiters. *Today's Health*, 51: (October, 1973).
35. _____: The Victimizing of Desperate Cancer Patients, *Today's Health*, 51: (November, 1973).
36. Seizures and Postal Service Cases, *FDA Consumer*, 9:33, (September, 1975).
37. _____. *FDA Consumer*, 9:32, (October, 1975).
38. _____. *FDA Consumer*, 9:36, (November, 1975).
39. _____. *FDA Consumer*, 9:37, (December, 1975-January, 1976).
40. Smith, Ralph Lee: *At Your Own Risk: The Case Against Chiropractic*. New York, Pocket Books, 1969.
41. Strovan, Clarence, *et al.* Community Nurse Practitioner—An Emerging Role. *American Journal of Public Health*, 64: (September, 1974).
42. United States Government Manual 1975/76: Washington, D.C., Government Printing Office, 1975, p. 500.
43. United States Department of Health, Education and Welfare: *Independent Practitioners Under Medicare—A Report to the Congress*. Washington, D.C., The Department, 1968.
44. _____: *Your Medicare Handbook*. Washington, D.C., Dept. of HEW, Social Security Administration, August, 1974.
45. *We Want You To Know About Today's FDA:* DHEW Pub. No. (FDA) 74-1021. Washington, D.C., Government Printing Office, 1974.
46. White, Carol: Medical Supplies You Should Always Have on Hand, *Today's Health*, 51: (January, 1973).

9

Your Choice—
Community Health

THE COMMUNITY-OF-SOLUTION AND YOU

You may tend to think of "community health" as encompassing a group of functions which are remote and irrelevant to the life and life-style of a college student. Often we think of community health as a something which is related to "others" and not ourselves, a something about which we can be concerned "later," or a something which concerns persons in lower socio-economic levels primarily. Actually, nothing could be further from the truth! Many agencies and groups cooperate to maintain the well-being of both large and small groups of people by surrounding them with what might be described as a large invisible shield of protection! And *you* are there in the middle of those small as well as large groups!

For example, how often do you stop to think about the purity of the drink that you take from a water fountain in the library or dining hall? Or how often do you question the contents of a can of juice or a square of chocolate from a candy bar or a cut of meat from a market? If each of these products appears to look and smell OK, you consume them with little question as to how they were processed and marketed. And cartons of milk are consumed with practically no thought or concern about pasteurization of all things!

By this time, you are realizing that community health and the purity of food, water, and milk are closely connected. And so are community health and cancer research, suicide prevention, poison control, and

158

venereal disease control. Although they contrast widely in scope, they all reflect a potential hazard or problem—to you and often to others. When, for one of a variety of reasons, the health of a segment of the community is in jeopardy, one of a variety of groups becomes concerned and tries to help. Or a group of concerned citizens rallies to form a group to meet the crisis or problem; citizens in the democracy of the United States of America are like that! Essentially, health is very much a community affair!

Actually, there are *many* invisible shields of protection around you—on the campus, on the highway, in your home town—which offer you many types of defense; their relevancy is *neither* a matter of choice or chance *and both* a matter of choice and chance. If you choose to live with others and not as a hermit in the United States today, the choice is not yours concerning many community protections; those in communes may or may not be affected, depending on where the commune is located. The matter of chance appears when you choose not to cooperate—i.e. on the highway or in disposing of garbage or in doing your own thing in such a way that you are an emotional or a social nuisance or hazard to others. This type of chance risks both your health and that of others and is not the intelligent type of risk discussed in Chapter 1.

Since most campuses are small communities in themselves, you are connected with community health and community health is connected with you in many ways every day. "Community health means the organized cooperative efforts of all agencies in the community directed toward the promotion of the physical, emotional and social health of the community residents."[8] The agencies involved may be numerous, or there may be a single structure, such as a University Health Center or Service. The agencies involved will be found on several levels—the university, local, or county level; the state or district level; and the national level. Some are international in scope. The agencies involved may have different functions in their mission of protecting your well-being—i.e., some offer you specific services, others tend to be primarily educational, while some focus on researching a particular problem or disease as their basic concern. Many organizations are involved in two or all of these functions. However, regardless of their specific function or on what "level" they operate, *you* as an individual member of a community of some type are their "raison d'etre."

Obviously, community health is as complex as the society which it serves. Since our contemporary life-style is overflowing with both social and physical complications, our community health structures do have their hands full—especially since they purport to serve all our health

needs—physical, social, emotional, and mental! And since communities
of persons vary in their needs and problems, there is no one structure or
group that can serve, educate, research, and then produce all the
necessary "solutions." The reasons for this are obvious—they are
economic, they are political, they are cultural and they are social
reasons in implication and nature. Thus, because our health needs are
myriad, we have many "communities-of-solution" so to speak. Or to put
it another way, different groups within the same or adjacent geographical areas have different types of health problems. Within a
community such as a Columbus, Ohio, or a South Bend, Indiana, or a
Greensboro, North Carolina, the university community contains certain
health concerns, while the urban area in that same community has other
problems which in turn are different from the concerns of the new
suburban developments. Thus, we have the so widely quoted concept of
community-of-solution identified in 1966 by The National Commission
on Community Health Services; this concept takes community health
out of its more traditional geographical identification or boundaries and
places it into "problem" identification or boundaries (that is, boundaries
"within which a problem can be defined, dealt with, and solved").[7] In
dissolving the "old" boundaries, a far greater arena is created within
which both the concepts of "community" and "health" are
extended—more problems are investigated and the scope of the concern
becomes far greater. To meet such a situation, more organizations and
agencies come onto the scene; obviously no one group has the "politic"
or finances to be able to cope with all communities and all solutions!
Thus, many types of groups on many different geographical levels
offering many different functions become important to you today as you
seek to find community health answers and make decisions.

   You may be asking—when does a personal health problem become
a health problem with community dimensions, or are all personal
health problems in reality problems which need to concern the community, also? Although no definitive "yes" or "no" can be assumed,
there are some general guidelines which might help answer this question. The most obvious discriminators would be those health problems
which affect a large number of people, such as an unusual number
of cases of measles in an elementary school or hepatitis on a university campus; the isolated case is usually an individual problem
unless it represents an extremely or potentially dangerous problem—
such as a case of smallpox in the United States would present today.
Another example would be a potentially dangerous curve in a highway
used by hundreds of commuters or a broken piece of concrete in steps in
a classroom building. A health problem may also assume community

characteristics when an individual is unable to cope because it necessitates large financial involvement—such as the use of an iron lung, a kidney machine, or extensive computer time. The community health problem rather than the personal one is present, also, when its solution requires the cooperation of a group of people—such as acquiring health insurance for the person who has epilepsy or combating misunderstanding about venereal disease treatment and prevention. And when the future well-being of a great many people is involved, as is the case today in many of our environmental problems, it becomes a problem of community proportions; an individual has a difficult time fighting the large manufacturing plant which is polluting the sky as well as the river. There is no one general rule-of-thumb guideline because of the complexity of our personal life-styles as well as the geographical, political, and cultural group differentials. You will be able to establish additional guidelines once you grasp the mix of the problems, the communities, the solutions and the variations in each!

A DIVERSITY OF PROBLEMS AND GROUPS

In order to meet such a diversity of problems in such diverse circumstances, we as a democratic people in these United States have created and endorse several different types of health agencies. They exist at varying levels, i.e. campus or local as a city or county, or state wide, or nation wide. Some exist at just one level (i.e. a local drug counseling center), while others are formed at all these levels—such as a "heart association" or "cancer society." Some even exist at an international level—such as The International Red Cross.

The manner in which these agencies are subsidized also varies. Those named in the preceding paragraph are all funded primarily through voluntary contributions, that is, via contributions from you and me as private citizens, memorials, bequests, or other fund-raising gimmicks. The ability of such organizations to even exist basically depends upon whether you and I want them to as evidenced by our willingness to support them financially. However, the solving of the health problems of communities cannot depend on adequate voluntary contributions. This is why the governmental or official health agency is of such major importance to the community scene and to us as individuals. The official agency receives its financial base from the process of taxation, whether from local (city or county), state, or federal taxes. As such, it is our representative and exists, theoretically, to serve us by protecting our health and helping prevent illness on both a personal and community scale.

Besides the voluntary and official (governmental) groups, there are others such as professional health organizations, (the American Medical Association and the American Dental Association); civic, youth-serving and fraternal groups such as Boy Scouts, Camp Fire Girls, Chamber of Commerce, and "Lions," who all have health as one of their several program objectives; plus various foundations (Ford Foundation, Rockefeller Foundation, and others) which also lend a hand in community health matters. No one group can do the total job, since maintaining and protecting the health of approximately 215 million people is a colossal task. It will never be possible, probably, to do it to the satisfaction or acclaim of most of the people in this country, since one's health behaviors and decisions are dependent upon so much more than a service being offered or a fact being known and accepted. Thus, the real issue becomes the identification of the health priorities and pertinent issues of a "community" and the extent to which they can be financed.

OFFICIAL HEALTH AGENCIES

The tasks which you often think about your own city health department undertaking are the traditional priorities such as collecting vital statistics, assuring pure water and pasteurized milk, and controlling diseases, especially communicable diseases. Gradually, however, as science and technology have simplifed and perfected these processes, as individuals have become aware of their importance, and as the standard of living in the United States has improved, the once traditional priorities have been able to be moved to the back burner in some communities. Since many public health experts feel that the number one public health problem today is *prevention*, many city and state health department roles will reflect preventive-type programs. The fundamentals of epidemiology are now being complemented by such programs as maternal and child health; dental health; mental health; alcoholism and drug addiction; mental retardation; prevention of chronic or noncommunicable disease; occupational health; disaster planning; accident prevention, and food and nutrition. The areas of environmental protection as well as consumer protection and control are also prominent. Once the basic fundamentals of communicable disease control and water and food purity are assured, each official agency at its own level within its financial capabilities incorporates as many of these features as feasible and as needed. Although some of the services are performed as "welfare actions" to those in medical need who are unable to pay, the majority of them in many communities are offered on an ability-to-pay scale.

Compiling vital statistics (including births, deaths and reportable diseases) is a program which has been and will continue to be a priority; it is an excellent example of one of several "common threads" or functions that may be found within all of the different levels of the official agencies, and which shows the interrelationship between the official agencies at the local, state, and national levels. Once the figures have been reported and collected from both the public and private sectors, they are computed and interpreted by the local authorities. Then they are sent to the state division of vital statistics. At this level, the statistics are again compiled as received from each local department and totaled for the state; then they are interpreted for the state as a whole. From the states they are sent to the National Center for Health Statistics where the same process is repeated from a national point of view.

Similar types of relationships of program function can be found in many programs with this same basic format. The grass roots of the programs are the local units—whether they be campus, city, or county based. This is where the action is! When the local unit cannot meet its basic needs, help may be sent from the state department of health in the form of consultation or money or personnel, if available. In general, state departments of health act as facilitators as well as coordinators for their local units. The same type of assistance is given them by the U.S. Department of Health, Education and Welfare, and specifically divisions within the Public Health Service. By means of funding or special grants, the federal government now gives direct financial assistance to both states and local communities to meet such personal challenges as alcoholism, drug abuse, and mental retardation via a "community" thrust.

As a socially conscious citizen, how do you fit into this picture? The key word here is *conscious!* Now you are aware that your campus health service does more than give flu shots and your home town health department does more than take chest x-ray films of food handlers or give dental care to low income patients. There are many services available to you which will improve your quality of life. Why not become acquainted with your health department—its budget may not make possible much wide scale advertising. Programs such as rape crises centers, venereal disease control and VD "Hotlines," suicide prevention, lead poisoning screening, genetic counseling, and nutrition for the elderly reflect some current local health department services. Some programs are organized and developed by local health department personnel who then train volunteers who staff them. Why not investigate yours? As a type of local health agency, the university health service may be able to answer many health needs that are beyond the control of you—the individual student.

Generally state departments of health do for the people of a state what their local departments cannot do—due to both financial and manpower reasons. Through their overall coordinating and political functions, they are able to assess the unmet needs or problems that local areas may be unable to do. A current organizational chart of a good sized state department is found in Figure 9-1.

The official health agency which we subsidize by our federal income taxes is a large complex organization known as the U. S. Department of Health, Education and Welfare. Although many taxpayers are unaware of its functions, they are essentially of value to know. If for no other reason, becoming acquainted with at least its major divisions will enable you to assess television and newspaper reports concerning federal health activities more accurately and knowledgably.

Under the leadership of the Secretary of HEW, a member of the Presidents' Cabinet, there are five major "working" divisions; these include:

1. Social Security Division
2. Social and Rehabilitation Service
3. Education Division
   a. Office of Education
   b. National Institute of Education (research oriented)
4. Office of Human Development
5. Public Health Service
   a. Food and Drug Administration
   b. National Institutes of Health
   c. Center for Disease Control
   d. Health Services Administration
   e. Health Resources Administration
   f. Alcohol, Drug Abuse, and Mental Health Administration

Of course, the division that is primarily concerned with "health" is the Public Health Service. However, some of the other divisions have definite health implications, as follows:

1. The *Social Security Division* has "insurance" as its key function, including, not only, retirement but also survivors, disability, and health insurance (Medicare) as discussed in Chapter 8; its programs serve people of all age groups.
2. The *Social and Rehabilitation Services* renders many health-related functions, including grants to states for programs that

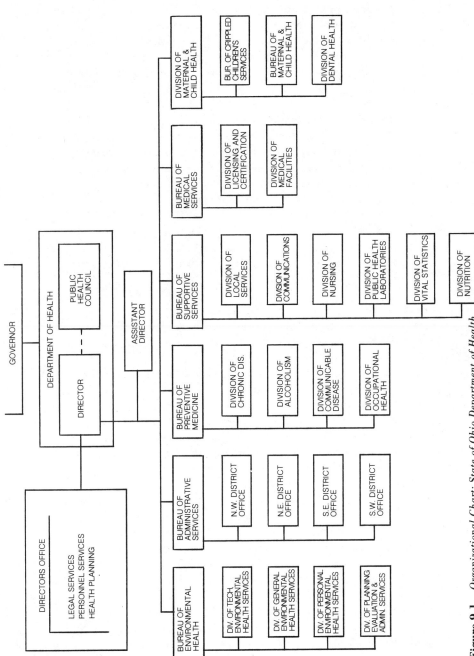

Figure 9-1. *Organizational Chart: State of Ohio Department of Health.*

provide medical services to the low income and the medical
needy. It also sponsors programs of vocational rehabilitation for
the disabled and for those with developmental disabilities.

3. The *Education Division* does not directly control the curricular
offerings of schools. This is done by individual states. Few
states can function independently, however, without federal
grants; these are distributed according to such factors as pupil
attendance, integration, and equal rights. This Division does
offer the funds for programs that individual states cannot
finance, including special Indian education, bilingual education, career education, and programs for the handicapped. The
National Institute of Education offers funds to groups to research special areas such as experimental schools and field
initiated studies.

4. The *Office of Human Development* is concerned with the
physical, social and emotional "rights" of many groups such as
the mentally retarded, the aged citizen, the youth in the inner
city, and the Native American.

The *Public Health Service* is, however, the major "health" facet
of the federal government at the national level. Although its five units
appear complex in an organizational chart, their functions can be
clearly identified and many have specific implications for you as a
student-citizen. The following information concerns a few selected
activities of each unit as they might concern you and is not intended
to completely delineate the functions of each.

Food and Drug Administration. As a consumer of health products
and services, the FDA forms an invisible shield of protection around
you in your purchase and use of drugs, foods, medical devices, toys,
imported goods, household chemicals and poisons, and cosmetics.
Its monthly periodical, The *FDA Consumer*, is written for the lay-
person and is most informative and enjoyable reading. There is one of
nineteen FDA District Offices near you to which you can report violations of the standards which are set for all these health products
and services. Chapter 8 further discusses its effectiveness regulations.

National Institutes of Health (NIH). This research arm of the
federal government is the major health researcher in the United
States today. Coordinated at its 300 acre campus in Bethesda, Mary-
land, the NIH actually consists of 10 separate Institutes including the
National Cancer Institute, National Heart and Lung Institute, National
Eye Institute, and National Institute of Neurological Disease and
Stroke, plus six others which focus on the major current problems of life

and death. At Bethesda there are patient facilities and services in a 500-bed hospital; here you may offer to enter a "healthy volunteer" program for a specified amount of time. A large number of the actual research projects are awarded to medical research facilities outside of NIH who then coordinates the results, many of which may culminate in actual treatment programs at the Clinical Center.

The *Center for Disease Control*, in directing national programs from Atlanta, Georgia, for the prevention and control of both communicable and non-communicable diseases, interprets and communicates to the public, as well as the states, the implications of contemporary disease problems, such as influenza, encephalitis, rubella, and other diseases from records and statistics. It also enforces foreign quarantine regulations when necessary, deploys a "medical detection" team when requested, has taken a leadership role in the problem of smoking and its relation to health and is focusing on effective methods of educating the general public via its Bureau of Health Education.

The *Health Services Administration* is primarily a service-oriented unit. It directs and/or funds health services for youth delinquency prevention, family planning groups, the Alaskan and American Indian reservations, maternal and child health units in states and cities, and many special community health projects.

The *Health Resources Administration* helps make available on either a direct or matching-fund basis additional health and medical facilities and personnel for communities. The Health Service building on your campus or the building which houses the health department in your home community may have been built with the aid of these funds. It is also concerned about health personnel and manpower and offers financial assistance to educational institutions of medical, dental, nursing, and allied health manpower to facilitate their curricula and to increase the number of qualified graduates in these areas.

The *Alcohol, Drug Abuse, and Mental Health Administration,* as a separate unit, reflects the severity of these problems in our life-style and culture today. This unit contains Institutes which research these problems, a few clinical centers which treat them, and clearinghouses which dispense the most up-to-date information and facts about these problems.

One of the major problems which the Congress of the United States is facing is the development of a system of national health insurance for people of all ages, not just for those over sixty years of age who are on Social Security. Several different plans are in the hopper as discussed in Chapter 8 and their formulation and legislation comprise one of the largest health issues in many years—large in terms of the necessary funding for appropriations and the impact of the controversy. The ramifications of whether the government should get into the health insurance business to such a large extent is a sensitive social and political issue regardless of the final decision.

Although the federal government pays the bill for a great many of the health services and much of the health research in this country, it does not, cannot, and probably never will be able to provide even minimal health care for thousands of individuals. Our health care system is partially based on the premise that the voluntary agencies and private foundations are going to offer a certain percent of support for specific client care and research of special health problems.

VOLUNTARY ORGANIZATIONS AND "GIVING"

The names of many of the voluntary health agencies in the United States today are common household terms—The American National Red Cross, The American Cancer Society, The American Heart Association and The American Lung Association (formerly The National Tuberculosis and Respiratory Disease Association). One of the reasons that we are so familar with these organizations is that they exist on all the "geographical" levels for many of us. We are aware that the "local" group sponsors many fund-raising events such as walkathons, balloon sales, seal sales, a special day-at-the-races, emergency drives, and other such events. We are aware, also, of the advertisements in newspapers and magazines as well as the 30-second public relations releases or "spots" on televisions on their behalf. The high degree of organization from the national level through the local unit has guaranteed funds totaling more than $30 million a year for each of several of these groups. They have spent money to become visible in order to raise money, and we as citizens have responded in large numbers to their appeals for several interesting reasons. The list of these prominent voluntary groups also includes the National Foundation (March of Dimes), National Association for Mental Health, National Easter Seal Society for Crippled Children and Adults and the Muscular Dystrophy Association of America, among others.

We have responded, too, to appeals of groups, perhaps lesser known nationally, but prominent and active such as the local or state Epilepsy Association, Arthritis Foundation, Leukemia Society, or Society for the Prevention of Blindness whose cause and needs are just as viable and just as great. In general, all of these voluntary health organizations are requesting contributions for several purposes. They are attempting to meet the specific needs of their clients through *services,* such as providing transportation to clinics or hospitals for treatment; self-help and therapeutic devices; job procurement counseling; medication; and socializing and recreational opportunities. They further attempt to *educate* the client, the general public, and other professionals about their special problem through films, literature, forums, etc. Finally, an effort is made by these groups if possible to further *research* and clarify the problem (i.e. find the cause of cancer).

Most of these groups have rung our doorbells or stopped us in the shopping centers or contacted us via the postal system with their individual appeals for donations. But we cannot overlook that there is the united or federated fund-raising appeal, known usually as the United Way or Community Chest, which represents a composite of many community agencies, of which health agencies may play a major part. The organizations which comprise the United Way (which may total as many as 40 to 50 in some communities) band together and work together in raising one large budget on a comprehensive basis in a comprehensive campaign; a small paid executive staff coordinates the one fund drive. Prior to the drive, each of the participating groups submits its budget and its proposed program which purports to eliminate duplicate services within a given community setting. In many cities the United Way campaign is the only one which is allowed to go directly into industrial and manufacturing plants and professional institutions to ask for contributions, which in turn can be deducted directly from a pay check if desired. Some large United Way campaigns even have executives from large and prominent manufacturers, banks, insurance companies, and other business loaned for the "United Way month" to facilitate public relations and fund raising activities within the community and its solicitors. Since the amount raised must be divided among all the groups participating according to prior appropriation decisions made by a committee of volunteer business and professional persons, most of the large (independent) voluntary groups do not participate in United Way. Some of their national organizations do not allow the local affiliates to do so; most of the others can raise far more on their own than they can "in concert" with the many other groups with which they would have to share. In 1913 when the federated type of giving was initiated, it was hoped that all fund raising groups in a community would join. This would, among other things, minimize the cost and time involved in fund raising, eliminate the annoying frequent requests for donations, reduce the confusion about organizations, and provide a more balanced consistent pattern of giving for many individuals. (Organizations within a United Way cannot further solicit funds on their own door to door.)

However, "individual rights" could not be served in this way for a variety of people and reasons. Thus, in most communities we have a United Way campaign as well as numerous independent agency fund-raising activities. You and I must make our own decisions as to how to divide our dollar(s) among these many groups.

This suggests that we must become wise givers since the majority of us may not feel we can purchase from every Boy Scout, Camp Fire Girl, Girl Scout, Band Booster, etc., etc., etc., that comes asking us to buy cards, chocolates, wrapping paper, etc., as well as reply positively to the solicitors for all those other voluntary organizations. Many of us may be unaware that the psychology used in requesting our help makes a lot of difference as to whether we give and how much. As a people, Americans are "soft-touches" in many ways and so we "give from the heart" rather than from a pre-thought-out pattern of giving. To that handsome little "cub scout" who rings your door bell, the cute little "Blue Bird" who wants you to help her go to camp and thus buy a can of hard candy, the friend who is soliciting the neighborhood for her favorite charity—for several reasons you may not feel you can or should say "no." The crippled child-of-the-year on the large billboards, the "poster person," the television personality who acts as the honorary chairman of the fund drive or who conducts the telethon—all of these are examples of fund raising psychology that is highly successful with many of us for obvious reasons! And when the "boss" asks you to give—you seldom say no, also! Then, there is the myriad of items that we receive through the mail—from minority groups, from handicapped persons, from orphanages, from displaced persons of many varieties—all requesting that we keep the plastic box or seals or cards or whatever and send a contribution to a given address! This type of solicitation is not unlawful, but if you did not request the item received in the mail you are under no obligation whatsoever to send it back, even if you choose not to contribute to the group; in most instances return postage is not guaranteed! Throw away the item if you cannot use it and do not wish to contribute to the organization. This type of mail solicitation is frowned upon by many voluntary organizations; it is expensive and contains little accountability about the organization per se. It costs money to raise money; fund raisers are cognizant of this and many groups tend to disguise these kinds of expenses under the heading of "public relations" or even public education, while others such as United Way are open about the amounts spent in fund-raising and proud of the fact that only a total of 9-10% of an annual budget is spent in this way.

In summary, knowing to whom to give and how much to give is too often an off-the-cuff decision! Planning ahead is helpful! You should also be aware of the fact that the telephone solicitor should be questioned carefully; the door-to-door bell ringers should have some type of identification proving that they do represent a bona fide local group, and give you a receipt for tax-deduction purposes. Since the majority of these groups do depend on individual door-to-door contributions for a certain percentage of their annual budgets, give your money to those that are important to you.

The "voluntary" agencies were so named for two basic reasons. When the majority of them were organized in the early 1900's or 1920-40's, they were dependent on voluntary contributions as the basic budget base as well as volunteer personnel to raise this money and also donate their time and skills to help achieve the organization's objectives. Volunteers spent time in association offices doing routine tasks and answering the telephone, working with clients, and fulfilling public information and public relations assignments. These groups operated on a volunteer-base, not a tax-generated base; however, this is also beginning to change to some extent. For purposes of tax exemption, each voluntary organization must be guided by a non-paid type of "Board of Trustees." This group makes the basic policies and decisions which in turn are carried out by a paid administrative staff. Since these groups are not accountable to us as people "of the whole" but rather to their constituents, voting members and donors, their programs can be flexible and sensitive to the needs of the group they are endeavoring to serve. More and more these Boards are appealing to the tax-subsidy agency and Foundations for monies for special projects which the bequests, memorials and door-to-door campaigns can no longer finance.

In general voluntary health agencies exist to "serve, educate and research" about (1) a specific disease entity such as the National Multiple Sclerosis Society or The American Diabetes Association; or (2) a specific structure or system of the human body, such as Pilot Dogs or the National Society for the Prevention of Blindness, or (3) a specific "people problem" such as the Planned Parenthood Federation of America or the American National Red Cross. The serving and educating is done basically in the local and state or district units, while the research is coordinated by a staff in the national headquarters. At one time much of the medical research was being conducted on grants from the voluntary associations; however, due to the rising costs of this activity and the coordination of it, plus the expanded entry of HEW into the research arena through the National Institutes of Health, the voluntary associations are no longer assuming the major research role. At this time, they work *with* NIH, not compete with it, in order to achieve the necessary medical break-throughs.

Research is still the principal function of some organizations such as the American Heart Association, the Leukemia Society of America, and the National Foundation (March of Dimes). The willingness of the federal government, as urged by the Congress, to try to solve the mysteries of cancer and drug abuse through the millions of dollars channeled into the National Cancer Institute and the Institute of Mental Health, is evidence of the major research role now being assumed by our national official health agency. Many voluntary agencies view this as a positive sign since it enables them to use their funds to better serve and educate the public.

PROFESSIONAL AND CIVIC GROUPS

There are many other groups beside the official and voluntary organizations that are our partners in our communities-of-solution! We cannot overlook (1) the civic and youth serving groups such as the Girl Scouts and Boy Scouts of America, the Camp Fire Girls, Inc., the 4-H Clubs, the Future Farmers of America, American Legion, YMCA and YWCA, and "J-C's"; (2) the fraternal groups such as the International Association of Lions Clubs, Kiwanis International, and Rotary International and; (3) the foundations, such as the Ford Foundation, the Kellogg Foundation, the Bronfman Foundation, and the Rockefeller Foundation which were established as a result of huge family and business fortunes. All of these groups play a part in enabling communities to cope with and meet problems; health of persons and communities is one of their program thrusts.

The professional health associations also have an indirect role to play in community health. Subsidized by individuals who qualify for membership by holding a specific license or certificate or diploma, these groups exist primarily to serve this membership. However, they also lend philosophical and psychological support as well as leadership to the basic concepts of community health, particularly those concerned with community health education. Such groups as the American Public Health Association, the Department of Health Education of the American Medical Association, the Association for the Advancement of Health Education, the American School Health Association, the Bureau of Dental Health Education of the American Dental Association and the National Safety Council are all examples of professional groups who contribute to the totality of community health.

YOUR ROLE—YOUR CHOICE

So, where do you fit into all this? You as a member of one or more communities-of-solution may be considered one of the most important constituents in this picture. *You* may be a leader of a community health cause, or an active worker, or a member of the silent majority. Regardless of how actively involved you become, you can fill two specific roles. In the first place you are a voting citizen and a tax payer as well as a payer of university tuition and fees; as such you have certain rights and responsibilities in health matters which you can accept or abdicate. You can be an effective extension of the Food and Drug Administration as well as your campus and local health departments by reporting health problems in place of ignoring them. Whether you want to make a choice of offering leadership, asking questions, and/or raising issues that concern the official agencies is up to you! Secondly, you are a socially conscious individual, and as a result of this chapter (hopefully), more conscious and more aware of voluntary organizations than you used to be! You can donate your time, your money, your blood, and/or your voice to many worthy health causes. You can be actively and directly *concerned* in many ways regardless of whether you contribute dollars and cents. You have skills which voluntary, civic, and youth serving groups need. The CHOICE is yours—do *not* leave it to chance and thus, perhaps, to non-solution!

PROBLEMS FOR YOUR CONSIDERATION

1. Discuss why the local health department is considered the "grass roots" of official health organizations. Then trace several of its major activities through your state department of health and the Department of Health, Education and Welfare.

2. Investigate various ways in which each of us can become an extension of the FDA.

3. Select one of the following health charity fund-raising approaches and then give the rationale for your choice:
   a. There should be just one united or federated type of fund-raising.
   b. All fund-raising should be conducted as independent enterprises (i.e., no "United Way").

c. There should be a coordinated combination of these philosophies and approaches.

4. Develop a series of "guidelines for wise giving" to voluntary health organizations and other health charities.

5. Identify the groups in your community who offer various types of crises-oriented assistance to citizens.

6. The Environmental Protection Agency is prominent on the national scene; investigate what state and local groups, both official and voluntary, are active in this concern in your community.

REFERENCES

1. Anderson, C. L.: *Community Health.* 2nd ed., St. Louis, The C. V. Mosby Co., 1973.
2. Asbell, Bernard: Good Volunteers Mind Other People's Business. *Today's Health* 53: (October, 1975).
3. Carter, Richard: *The Gentle Legions.* New York, Doubleday and Company, Inc. 1961.
4. *Directory of Services:* Columbus (Ohio) Health Department, Columbus, The Department, n.d.
5. Gildea, William: Children's Charities: The Golden Fleece? *Today's Health* 52: (October, 1974).
6. Grant, Murray: *Handbook of Community Health.* 2nd Ed., Philadelphia, Lea & Febiger, 1975.
7. *Health Is a Community Affair:* Report of the National Commission of Community Health Services. Cambridge, Mass., Harvard University Press, 1966, p. 2.
8. Henkel, Barbara Osborn: *Community Health.* 2nd Ed., Boston, Allyn and Bacon, Inc., 1970, p. 3.
9. Katz, Harvey: *Give! Who Gets Your Charity Dollar?* New York, Anchor Press/Doubleday, 1974.
10. McTaggart, Aubrey C.: *The Health Care Dilemma.* Boston, Holbrook Press, Allyn and Bacon, Inc., 1971, 127-161.
11. Wigley, Richard and Cook, James R.: *Community Health Concepts & Issues.* New York, D. Van Nostrand Company, 1975.
12. *United States Government Manual 1975/76:* Office of the Federal Register. Washington, D.C., Government Printing Office. 1975, 221-254.
13. *Wise Giving Bulletin:* (A Reporting and Advisory Service for Contributors) New York, National Information Bureau, Inc. Quarterly.

Index

Page numbers in *italics* refer to illustrations; page numbers followed by "t" refer to tables.